Perl Programming
for Biologists

Perl Programming for Biologists

D. Curtis Jamison

Center for Biomedical Genomics and Informatics
George Mason University
Manassas, Virginia

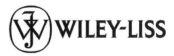

A JOHN WILEY & SONS, INC., PUBLICATION

For general information on our other products and services please contact our Customer Care
Department within the U.S. at 877-762-2974, outside the U.S. at 317-572-3993 or fax 317-572-4002.

Wiley also publishes its books in a variety of electronic formats. Some content that appears in
print, however, may not be available in electronic format.

Library of Congress Cataloging-in-Publication Data:

Jamison, D. Curtis.
   Perl programming for biologists / D. Curtis Jamison.
      p. cm.
Includes bibliographical references (p.   ).
   ISBN 0-471-43059-5(Paper)
   1. Biology – Data processing. 2. Perl (Computer program language) I.
Title.
   QH324.2 .J36 2003
   570′.28′55133 – dc21

                                             2002152547

Printed in the United States of America.

10 9 8 7 6 5 4 3 2 1

Contents

Perl Programming for Biologists,   D. Curtis Jamison
ISBN 0-471-43059-5   Copyright © 2003 Wiley-Liss, Inc.

Part I

The Basics

Introduction

Molecular biology is a study in accelerated expectations.

In 1973, the first paper reporting a nucleotide sequence derived directly from the DNA was reported. During the late 1970s, a graduate student could earn a Ph.D. and publish multiple papers in *Science, Cell*, or any number of respected journals by performing the astonishing task of sequencing a gene – any gene. By 1982, DNA sequencing had become straightforward enough that any well-equipped laboratory could clone and sequence a gene, providing they had a copy of *Molecular Cloning: A Laboratory Manual.* By 1990, simply sequencing a gene was considered sufficient for only a master's degree, and most journals considered the sequence of a gene to be only the starting point for a scientific paper. The last sequencing-only paper published was the full genomic sequence of an organism. By 1995, the majority of journals had stopped publishing sequence data completely. In 1999, mid-way through the Human Genome Sequencing Project, approximately 1.5 megabases of human genomic sequence were being deposited in GenBank monthly, and by the end of 2001 there were almost 15 billion bases of sequence information in the databases, representing over 13 million sequences.

Bioinformatics, by necessity, is following the same growth curve.

Once a rarified realm, computers in biology have become common place. Almost every biology lab has some type of computer, and the uses of the computer range from manuscript preparation to Internet access, from data

Perl Programming for Biologists, D. Curtis Jamison
ISBN 0-471-43059-5   Copyright © 2003 Wiley-Liss, Inc.

collection to data crunching. And for each of these activities, some form of bioinformatics is involved.

The field of bioinformatics can be split into two broad fields: computational biology and analytical bioinformatics. Computational biology encompasses the formal algorithms and testable hypotheses of biology, encoded into various programs. Computational biologists often have more in common with people in the campus computer science department than with those in the biology department, and usually spend their time thinking about the mathematics of biology. Computational biology is the source of the bioinformatic tools like BLAST or FASTA, which are commonly used to analyze the results of experiments.

If computational biology is about building the tools, analytical bioinformatics is about using those tools. From sequence retrieval from GenBank to performing an analysis of variance regression using local statistical software, nearly every biological researcher does some form of analytical bioinformatics. And just as DNA sequencing has turned into a Red Queen pursuit, every biology researcher has to perform more and more analytical bioinformatics to keep up.

Fortunately, keeping up is not as hard as it used to be. The explosion of the Internet and the use of the World Wide Web (WWW) as a means of accessing data and tools means that most researchers can keep up simply by updating the bookmarks file of their favorite browser. In itself, this is no mean feat – Internet research skills can be tricky to acquire and even trickier to understand how to use properly. Still, there is a way to go further: one can begin to manipulate the data returned from conventional programs.

Data manipulation can usually be done in spreadsheets and databases. Indeed, these two types of programs are indispensable in any laboratory, especially those quite sophisticated in analytical bioinformatics. But to take the final step to truly exploit data analysis tools, a researcher needs to understand and be able to use a scripting language.

A scripting language is similar in most ways to a programming language. The user writes computer code according to the syntactic conventions of the language, and then executes the result. However, a scripting language is typically much easier to learn and utilize than a traditional programming language, because many of the common functions people use have already been created and stored. Additionally, most scripting languages are interpreted (turned into binary computer instructions on the fly) rather than compiled (turned into binary computer instructions once), so that scripts development is generally quicker and the scripts themselves are more portable.

Of course, there is always a price to pay for things being easier, and in the case of scripting languages, the major price is speed. Scripting languages typically take longer to execute than compiled code. But, except for the most extreme cases, the trade-off for ease of use over speed is quite acceptable, and might not even be noticeable on the faster computers available today.

The Perl programming language is probably the most widely used scripting language in bioinformatics. A large percentage of programs are written in Perl, and many bioinformatists cut their programming teeth using Perl. In fact, the most common advice heard by aspiring bioinformatists is "go learn Perl."

In part, Perl is a popular language because it is less structured than traditional programming languages. With fewer rules and multiple ways to perform a task, Perl is a language that allows for fast and easy coding. For the same reasons, it is an easier language to learn as a first programming language. But the very ease of using Perl is a bit of a trap: it is quite easy to make simple mistakes that are difficult to catch.

But there are strong reasons to learn and use Perl. The language was originally created for parsing files and quickly creating formatted reports. Larry Wall, the author of Perl, claims the name stands for "Practical Extraction and Reporting Language" (but he acknowledges that the name could just as easily stand for "Pathologically Eclectic Rubbish Lister") and the language is perfect for rummaging through files looking for a particular pattern of characters, or for reformatting data tables. The program has a very powerful regular expression capability for pattern matching, as well as built-in file manipulation and input/output (I/O) piping mechanisms. These abilities have proven invaluable for bioinformatics, where we are often looking for motifs within sequences (pattern-matching) or rearranging one database format into another.

The biggest use of Perl is the quick and dirty creation of small analysis programs. Nearly every bioinformatist has written a program to parse a nucleotide sequence into the reverse complement sequence. Similarly, a great many people use small Perl scripts to read disparate data files and parse the relevant data into a new format. This usage is so prevalent that the term "glutility" was coined by Sam Cartinhour for scripts that take the output of one program (like BLAST, for example) and change it into a form suitable for import into another program (like ClustalW). Finally, with the advent of the WWW, Perl has become the language of choice to create Common Gateway Interface (CGI) scripts to handle form submissions and create compute servers on the WWW.

The purpose of this book is to teach you Perl programming. What sets this book apart from most Perl language books is 1) the assumption that you've never had any formal training in programming, and 2) the examples are geared toward real problems biologists face, so you don't have to either learn an entirely new concept to understand the example or wrestle with an example that is generic and difficult to extrapolate into the real world of the laboratory.

At the conclusion of the book, you should be able to write a script to fix the clone library prefix that your summer student mistyped on every line of the spreadsheet, or to scan a Fasta sequence file for every occurrence of an EcoRI site. Moreover, you'll be able to write reusable and maintainable scripts so you don't have to rewrite the same piece of code over and over. Additionally, you'll be able to look at other people's scripts and adapt them to your own purposes. After all, to quote Larry Wall, the creator of Perl, "For programmers, laziness is a virtue."

Chapter 1

An Introduction to Perl

1.1   The Perl Interpreter

Computer programs are a set of instructions that tell the computer how to move electrons around inside. Computers operate in a binary manner, that is, any given memory spot is either a 0 or a 1. Each spot that can hold a 0 or 1 is known as a bit. The patterns of bits that are passed to the central processor unit determine exactly what the program does.

The earliest computers were programmed by inputting the patterns of 0's and 1's directly by flipping toggle switches. Later, when easier methods of inputting a program (like punch cards) were invented, people invented mnemonics to stand in for specific bit patterns and created programs called assemblers to translate the mnemonic code into a set of binary instructions. Later still, people created compilers that could understand more complex code than assemblers. Computer languages proliferated, with arcane languages springing up wherever there was a specialized need.

Into this landscape of specialized and complex computer programs came Perl, a generalized language that is relatively simple yet still very powerful. Perl programs are not compiled into binary code. Rather, they are interpreted when the program is launched, avoiding the need for a separate compilation step. Interpreted programs run almost as quickly as compiled programs, but are much easier to develop and alter.

Perl Programming for Biologists,   D. Curtis Jamison
ISBN 0-471-43059-5   Copyright © 2003 Wiley-Liss, Inc.

Perl programs are often referred to as scripts, because they are loaded into the Perl interpreter at runtime. The implication of this strategy is that you must have a Perl installation on your computer: a Perl script without an interpreter is simply an oddly formatted text file.

Fortunately, Perl interpreters are available for almost every operating system in existence, and typically come as a standard package under most versions of Unix (including the new Mac OS X). The latest version of Perl for any computer and the instructions on how to install it can always be found at the official Perl website (http://www.perl.org). The actual mechanisms of running Perl scripts are different for each operating system, so this section (and the book in general) focuses on generic Unix instructions, and on non-Unix systems your actual mileage may vary. Also, a general appreciation of how to use the Unix command line will be useful as you progress through the book.

1.2   Your First Perl Program

The best way to learn Perl is by doing it, so without further explanation, let's jump into a program. Traditionally, the first program anyone writes in a language is called "Hello world," where you make the computer print out the message. Perl allows us to do this using the print function. The simplest form of the print function takes a single argument and writes it to the standard output device, which is (usually) the terminal window on our computer screen. So our script will consist of one simple statement:

```
print "Hello world!\n";
```

We'll use this little program to illustrate how to run a Perl script.

There are two ways to start a Perl script running. In the first method, the Perl interpreter can be invoked as a normal program from the command line. A text file containing a Perl script is given to the interpreter as a Unix command line argument. So, as a first step we need to create a script file. Use your favorite text editor[1] to create a file called "hello.pl" that contains the following two lines:

```
# a silly script to output text
print "Hello world!\n";
```

Note that we included a comment line that explains what the program does. Although trivial in this example, it is a good idea to put a comment block at the beginning of every program that identifies what the program does, what arguments the program takes, who wrote it, and when it was written. This practice saves lots of time when you have a directory full of Perl scripts and you're not quite sure which one does what.

---

[1]There is a difference between text editors and word processors. Text editors create files containing only ASCII characters, whereas word processors embed hidden formatting codes that will confuse the Perl interpreter.

Run the program from the Unix command line by invoking Perl with the name of the file:

```
% perl hello.pl
Hello world!
```

The interpreter did exactly what the script asked it to do. It took the Perl statement, interpreted it, and then executed it. Note that the print statement only printed out what was between the double quotes: the quotes turn the phrase "Hello world!\n" into a character string with a line return at the end. Character strings are covered in more detail in the next chapter.

The most common way to start a Perl script is to make the script self-executable using the Unix command shell system. First, a special line must be inserted at the beginning of the script to tell Unix to use the Perl interpreter to run the script. The line begins with the characters "#!" followed by the command to start the Perl interpreter. Second, we need change the Unix permissions mask associated with the file. Use the chmod command to set the file to executable (for more information, type "man chmod" at the Unix prompt). Now the Perl script can be run from the Unix command line by typing the name of the Perl script (and any command line arguments your program needs).

To make our program easier to use, let's make this script self-contained. Edit the hello.pl file and put a line at the beginning that reads "#! /usr/bin/perl" (substitute the full and proper path to your Perl installation: if you're not sure where it is, type "which perl" at the command line and Unix will tell you the path). The entire program file should now look like

```
#! /usr/bin/perl
# a silly script to output text
print "Hello world!\n";
```

The "#!" combination of characters at the beginning of the script tells Unix that the code needs to be run by a particular script interpreter, and Unix command processor takes care of properly invoking the interpreter specified and hands the rest of the script file off to the interpreter.

Now we need to make the program executable by typing "chmod +x hello.pl" at the command line. Once the program is marked as executable, you can run it by simply typing in the file name:

```
%hello.pl
Hello world!
```

Congratulations! You're now a Perl programmer. All that's left now are some minor details, which we'll cover in the rest of the book.

1.3   How the Perl Interpreter Works

The first thing Perl does with the script is to read it and turn it into a machine-executable binary (*e.g.*, Perl interprets the script). During this process, Perl watches for syntax errors, which are places where it can't make sense of the script. Usually these are typos or the wrong number of arguments passed to a subroutine. If errors are found, Perl issues an error statement indicating where it got confused and why, and then exits to the Unix prompt. Otherwise, Perl begins to feed instructions to the CPU to run the script.

There are a couple of very nice things that the interpreter does for you when you run a script. First, it strips out any extra blank spaces and lines that are found in the code. This allows you to write the script formatted in a manner that makes it easier to see what is going on. Second, the compiler strips out any part of a line following the # symbol. The # symbol indicates that the following text to the end of the line is a comment, allowing you to insert small pieces of explanation, which is invaluable when you are trying to remember exactly what a complex section of code does six months or a year after you wrote it.

The behavior of the Perl interpreter can be controlled using command-line switches. A command line switch is a minus sign followed by a letter. The most commonly used command line switch is the – w switch that turns on the warnings and has Perl issue copious messages about statements that might cause problems. Switches can be added at the end of the #! line.

The structure of a Perl script is very simple. A script consists of a series of statements. A statement is a Perl command or function and associated arguments, and is terminated by a semicolon. In our first program, we had one statement consisting of the print function and a single argument telling Perl what to print, with the semicolon at the end. Although most people put one statement per line, Perl actually doesn't care and will quite happily interpret a statement that is spread across multiple lines or concatenated with several others on one line.

Statements can be grouped into code blocks using the curly braces { and } to delineate the beginning and the end of the code block, respectively. Code blocks will become very important in Chapter 4, when we talk about Perl commands that control whether or not some of our statements get run or not. Code blocks can also be used to make our program more readable.

There are almost as many styles of writing Perl code as there are Perl programmers. The choice of what style to follow is strictly up to the programmer, but some style conventions format code in a logical and readable way so you or someone else can look at it in the future and easily understand what the code does without digging through miles of spaghetti. I'll teach by example by formatting all the example code in the book using a standard format (one that I require my own students to follow).

Chapter Summary

- Perl is an interpreted scripting language.
- Scripts can be run from the command line or as a self-executable command.

- A # sign signifies a comment, and hides the rest of the line.

- A statement is always terminated by a semicolon.

For More Information

A quick note on the convention here: Books are given in standard citation form. The two books listed here, *Learning Perl* and *Programming Perl*, are the basic bibles for Perl programmers, and are valid as entries for all future chapters.

Schwartz, R. L. and Phoenix, T. (2001) *Learning Perl*, 3rd *Ed.* O'Reilly and Associates, Sebastapol, CA (www.oreilly.com).

Wall, L., Christiansen, T. and Orwant, J. (2000) *Programming Perl*, 3rd *Ed.* O'Reilly and Associates, Sebastapol, CA (www.oreilly.com).

The Perl documentation is rich and wonderful. The main help program is a perlscript called perldoc. Giving perldoc an argument will make it page out all the information it knows on the subject. The relevant perldoc references are given here, as a line to type at the command line. The first apparently redundant command given here is a way to get more information about the perldoc script itself, the second is more information about how Perl works.

```
perldoc perldoc
perldoc perlrun
```

Exercises

1. What is the path to your Perl installation?

2. Explain the difference between a compiler and an interpreter.

3. Classify the Perl switches given in the perlrun perldoc into two groups: those that are useful for running a script from the command line and those that are useful in the #! line for self-executing scripts (note that some switches may be useful in both groups). Explain your groupings.

4. When is it useful to make a script self-executable? When is it not necessary?

5. Which of the following lines look like valid Perl script commands, and which are likely to cause problems?

```
print "Hello World\n";
print "Helloworld\n";
print "Hello World"\n;
print "Hello World\n"
print "Hello World\n"; #
print #"Hello World\n";
#print "Hello World\n";
```

Chapter 2

Variables and Data Types

2.1 Perl Variables

In the early 1980's George Carlin had a comedy routine about how all he really needed was a place for his stuff. That sentiment is true for computer programs as well. It is the job of a programmer to create nice places to store stuff for the program, where things can easily be put away or retrieved. The stuff for a program is of course the data, and the nice places are variables.

A variable is a named reference to a memory location. Variables provide an easy handle for programmers to keep track of data stored in memory. In fact, we typically don't know the exact value of what is in a particular memory location, but rather we know the general type of data that could be stored there.

Perl has three basic types of variables. Scalar variables hold the basic building blocks of data: numbers and characters. Array variables and hash variables hold lists, and we'll discuss these variables in detail in Chapter 3. The three types are differentiated by the first character in the variable name: '$', '@', and '%', respectively. Following the type symbol, the name can be practically any combination of characters and of arbitrary length. Creating a variable is as simple as making up a variable name and assigning a value to it.

There are some rules associated with creating names. First and foremost, the second character of a name should be either a letter (A to Z or a to z), a digit (0 to 9), or an underscore (_). You can create variable names that don't adhere to this rule and begin with an obscure punctuation mark like ! or ?, but in this

Perl Programming for Biologists,   D. Curtis Jamison
ISBN 0-471-43059-5   Copyright © 2003 Wiley-Liss, Inc.

Table 2.1   Valid and invalid variable names

Variable Name	Comment
$a	valid
$apple_g4_computer_counter	valid: names can be any length with most alpha numeric characters
$my invalid variable name	invalid: spaces are one type of characters which aren't allowed (use underscores)
$my(invalid[variable{name}])	invalid: parens, brackets, and braces are allowed, but do something different that you might be intending (see Chapter 3)
$1 through $9	valid: "special" reserved variables
$_	valid: "special" reserved variable

case the variable name is limited to that character only. Most variable names that consist of a single character have a predefined significance to Perl, and you should avoid tromping on them (see Section 2.6).

The second variable naming rule says names that have a digit in the second position can only contain more digits, whereas names with a letter or an underscore have no restrictions. So if you were to create a variable named $100, you could not name a related variable $100a. Table 2.1 shows some examples of valid and invalid variable names.

Finally, it is useful to remember that variable names are case-sensitive. This means that $cat refers to a different spot of memory than $CAT.

Assigning a value to a variable is even easier than creating a name. All you have to is write an equation, with the variable name on the left, an = sign, and the value on the left. The = symbol is often called the assignment operator, because it is used to assign a value to a variable.

2.2   Scalar Values

Perl has two basic types of scalar values: numbers and strings. Both types can be assigned to a scalar variable.

Numbers are specified in any of the common integer or floating point formats:

```
$y = 1;          # integer
$x = 3.14;       # floating point
$w = 2.75E-6;    # scientific/engineering notation
$t = 0377;       # octal
$u = 0xffff;     # hexadecimal
```

The integer and floating point examples are standard enough, but the final three might look a little odd to computer novices. Numbers expressed in scientific notation are typically written as a floating point number times a power of 10. So, in a book, you would find the number written out as 2.75×10^{-6}. However, computers don't understand superscript, and Perl strips out the white spaces, so

2.75×10^{-6} becomes $2.75 \times 10 - 6$ and now we can't tell the difference between a very small number and an equation directing the computer to subtract 6 from the product of 2.75 and 10. So the engineering notation was invented simply by replacing the "$\times 10$" with "E" and putting the power on the same line.

The final two representations are numbers in nondecimal bases that don't occur often in bioinformatic programs, but occasionally crop up in compressed file formats (*e.g.*, ABI trace files are stored in hexadecimal). Octal is base 8, and hexadecimal is base 16, which are 2^3 and 2^4, respectively, and Perl allows programmers to use those numbers directly.

A string is a group of characters strung together, enclosed by quotation marks (the quotes can be either single or double quotes, but the choice does make a difference as we will see shortly). The characters can be any symbol available in the character set. Additionally, there are some special double character codes defined for text formatting, of which the two most important ones are "\n", which is the newline character, and "\t", which is the tab character. We have already seen the newline character in our hello.pl program.

Recall our program from Chapter 1. In that program, we asked Perl to print the phrase `"Hello world!"` for us. The phrase is actually a string, and we can assign the string to a variable. Furthermore, we can provide that variable to the print function, just like it was the string itself. So we can take our original hello.pl file:

```
#! /usr/bin/perl
# a silly script to output text
print "Hello world!\n";
```

and alter it to contain a variable:

```
#! /usr/bin/perl
# a silly script to output text
$string = "Hello world!\n";
print $string;
```

When you run the program again, you should see the same result as before:

```
%hello.pl
Hello world!
```

There are a few things to note from this example. First, to create and use a variable we simply create a variable name ($string) and assign a value (`"Hello world!\n"`) to it. Second, we can now use the new variable as if it were the value itself; that is, we can pass $string to the print function as if it were the string itself and Perl understands that we don't want to print the variable name but rather the value contained in the $string variable.

Finally, note that the program is executed sequentially, starting at line one and progressing line by line. First we assign a value to the $string variable, then we print the value contained in $string. This step-by-step progression through the script ensures that we can properly prepare all the variables for use (in this case assigning the value to the variable before we print).

Strings are typically used to contain words and sentences. They can also be used to store things like the character representation of a DNA segment or a protein. In fact, Perl has extremely powerful string manipulation capabilities that make it simple to create bioinformatic tools that find motifs, translate DNA sequences to RNA, or transcribe RNA sequences to protein. The string manipulation routines are explored in more detail in Chapter 6.

Because numbers and strings are both valid scalar values, it doesn't matter to Perl which type of value is stored in the variable. Numbers and strings can be stored interchangeably in the same variable:

```
#! /usr/bin/perl
# example of scalar values

$var = 29;
$var = "dog";
$var = 5;
$var = "cat";
```

is a perfectly valid script, since each of the values is a valid scalar value.

In fact, Perl will automatically convert from one type of scalar to another. For example, if we assign a numeric value to a variable, and then pass that variable to the print function, the number is converted automatically to a string:

```
#! /usr/bin/perl
# example of scalar values

$var = 29;
print $var;
```

which will print the same thing as

```
#! /usr/bin/perl
# example of scalar values

$var = "29";
print $var;
```

Both programs will print a '2' character followed by a '9' character.

Going in the other direction, Perl will attempt to convert a string to a number when it is used in a context where a number is required. The conversion proceeds from left to right, and stops as soon as Perl encounters a character that isn't part of a number. So, in the following example,

```
$x = "123";
$y = "50%";
$z = "cow5";
```

each of the variables would be translated as best as possible in a numeric context. The first, $x would have the value of 123, while the second would have the value of 50 in a numeric context. The final example $z would end up with a value of 0 in a numeric context: even though it contains the number 5 the first character is a 'c' that can't be translated.

It is important to note that the attempt at conversion does not change the original value of the variable. After the code snippet

```
$number = 29;
$string = "5dog";
$sum = $number+ $string;
```

is run, the value in $string is still "5dog" even though Perl converted it to the number 5 temporarily in order to add it to the value stored in $number.

2.3 Calculations

Because we have numbers, it would be quite useful to be able to do some mathematics with them. All the usual arithmetic operators from high school math are available to be used, and a few others that might be a surprise. Many of the available operators are listed in Table 2.2.

The mathematical operations are performed in the standard order of precedence that we all learned in grade school. For example, multiplication has a higher precedence than addition, so it gets done first:

$$2 + 3 * 4$$

is equal to 24, not 20. To make the equation evaluate to 20, we need to include parentheses to group together the step(s) we want to do first:

$$(2 + 3) * 4$$

tells Perl to sum the 2 and 3 first, even though the multiplication has a higher precedence.

Operators with the same precedence, like add and subtract, get done going from left to right. However, the cardinal rule to follow is to add parentheses

Table 2.2 Perl operators

++	Autoincrement
−−	Autodecrement
**	Exponentiation
*	Multiply
/	Divide
%	Modulus
+	Add
−	Subtract
cos()	Cosine
sin()	Sine
sqrt()	square root
=	Assign
+=	assign add
−=	assign subtract

whenever an equation is getting too tough to follow. That way, the real sense of what you are trying to do comes through. In many of the following examples, the parentheses are not strictly necessary, but are added to improve readability.

Most of the operators work on either bare numbers or upon the value stored in a variable. If the value is a string value that can be converted to a number, that conversion takes place first. Otherwise, the value is treated as a 0.

The first group of operators works solely upon variables. The autoincrement and autodecrement operators increase and decrease the variable by one, respectively. So if $a contains the value 1, after the statement

```
$a++;
```

$a contains the value 2. The operators can be placed either in front of or behind the variable, but the placement does make a difference in meaning. If the operator is placed after the variable, the increment is performed after the rest of the expression has been evaluated. If placed before the variable, the increment is performed before evaluation. This will make a big difference later in the book, when we are evaluating expressions as controls for loops; just store it away someplace in your gray cells for the moment.

The exponentiation operator takes the left operand and raises it the power of the right operand. Thus

```
$j = 2**3;        # $j = 8
```

means 2^3.

Perl can handle negative bases and negative exponents. It can also handle nonintegral exponents if the base is positive. Like most of us, Perl has trouble with complex and imaginary numbers, and special Perl libraries called modules need to be installed to deal with them (Chapter 8 explains modules in detail).

The multiplicative and additive operators are exactly what you would expect: they work on numbers to add, subtract, multiply, and divide. Some people might not have seen the modulus operator before: it returns the remainder from a divide operation:

```
$j = 52%3;        # $j = 1
```

The modulus operator determines the closest whole integer that the number on the right can generate, and then subtracts it from the number on the left and returns the result. In the example, the closest multiple of 3 is 51, so the modulus operator would calculate

```
52-(17*3)
```

and would return 1.

There are a number of named unary operators. A unary operator takes a number and return a calculated value. These also operate pretty much as one would expect:

```
$j = sqrt(2);            # $j = 1.4142135623731
```

The operand is given to the unary operator by enclosing it in parentheses immediately following the operator. As we will see in Chapter 5, this is very similar to the way we pass information to subroutines. In fact, unary operators can be considered a form of a subroutine.

Finally, the assignment operators put a value into a variable. We have been using the standard assignment operator all along: it looks like an equal sign and basically moves the value on the right into the variable on the left. It has the lowest precedence of any operator, because we want all the math complete before moving the value in place.

Perl also provides a large number of shortcut assignment operators. These are used to write things in shorthand. Perl interprets statements written

```
$var OP = $value
```

as

```
$var = $var OP $value
```

Thus,

```
$j += 1;
$j = $j +1;
```

both mean the same thing: add 1 to the value in $j. It is just that the former way of writing it can be a little clearer and a little quicker in some cases.

2.4   Interpolation and Escapes

When working with strings, the type of quotation mark around the string makes a difference as to how Perl treats it. A string enclosed in double quotes undergoes a process called interpolation, and anything that Perl recognizes as a variable gets replaced by the value of that variable. Let's alter hello.pl once again to illustrate interpolation:

```
#! /usr/bin/perl
# a silly script to output text
$string = "Hello world!\n";
print "The CONTENT of our variable is $string";
```

When we run this script, we get the following output:

```
% hello.pl
The CONTENTS of our variable is Hello world!
%
```

A string in single quotes is not interpolated, and any character in it is used exactly as is. Thus, if we wanted to print the name of a variable, we would pass it as a string encased in single quotes. For example, consider what happens when we use a single quote in the script:

```
#! /usr/bin/perl
# a silly script to output text
$string = "Hello world!\n";
print 'The NAME of our variable is $string';
```

When we run this script, we get the following output:

```
% hello.pl
The NAME of our variable is $string%
```

Because we are not interpolating the output string, we print it exactly as is without interpolating the $string variable.

One obvious difficulty with variable interpolation is how to embed special characters into an output. For example, we might want to exactly produce the line:

```
Today's "Blue-Plate Special" costs $5.99.
```

A simple print statement won't work:

```
print 'Today's "Blue-Plate Special" costs $5.99.'
```

produces an error message:

```
Unmatched '.
```

This is because Perl always matches an open quote with the first close quote it finds, which in this case is the hyphen in Today's. To deal with this, we can hide a character from Perl using the backslash character:

```
print 'Today\'s "Blue-Plate Special" costs $5.99.'
```

produces the requested line.

We refer to characters hidden by a backslash as backslash-escaped characters. In a single-quoted, noninterpolated string the only character that can be hidden is a single quote. A backslash in front of any other character is printed as is:

```
print 'Today\'s \"Blue-Plate Special\" costs $5.99.'
```

produces

```
Today's \"Blue-Plate Special\" costs $5.99.
```

Backslash-escaped characters are much more useful (and necessary) in double-quoted, interpolated strings. If we change our statement to an interpolated version:

```
print "Today\'s \"Blue-Plate Special\" costs $5.99."
```

the backslashes protect the single quote and the double quotes, but we get an odd result:

```
Today's "Blue-Plate Special" costs .99.
```

The $5 was interpolated as a variable. Because we didn't define $5 as a variable, the value of $5 was undef (nothing), and Perl printed nothing. Obviously we need to backslash-escape any dollar sign we want to print:

```
print "Today\'s \"Blue-Plate Special\" costs \$5.99."
```

Another important use for backslash-escaped characters is for special formatting characters. If you tried running some of the previous examples, you might have noticed a minor formatting problem:

```
haydn 10% Perl example_1
Today's "Blue-Plate Special" costs $5.99.haydn 11%
```

The Unix prompt for the next command appears on the same line as the output from the script. This is because the print function doesn't include the code for a new line. Look back at the Hello world! example script in the first chapter. At the end of the line, there is a backslash-escaped "n". This is the Unix convention for new line, which Perl adheres to. So, if we put a "\n" at the end of our print statement:

```
print "Today\'s \"Blue-Plate Special\" costs \$5.99.\n"
```

our output looks much better:

```
haydn 10% Perl example_1
Today's "Blue-Plate Special" costs $5.99.
haydn 11%
```

Perl has several special reserved backslash-escape codes, a partial list of which is shown in Table 2.3. These codes are very useful for formatting data. Beyond these codes, applying a backslash-escape to any other character interpolates to the character.

A special type of interpolation happens to strings enclosed by back ticks (accent grave). In this case, all the embedded variables are interpolated and the

Table 2.3 Special formatting character escapes

Character	Function
\n	new line
\t	Tab
\u or \U	force to upper case (one character or following characters)
\l or \L	force to lower case (one character or following characters)
\E	end \U or \L

string is passed to the system to be executed as a command. The differences between the three forms of quotations are illustrated in the following script:

```
#! /usr/bin/perl
# script to illustrate interpolation
$var = "ls  -l";   # the Unix command to print a directory listing
print '$var';
print "$var";
print '$var';
```

Despite the overt similarities, the three print statements produce three very different results. The first print statement writes out the string exactly as written:

```
$var
```

whereas the second print statement interpolates the string and replaces the $var variable with the value:

```
ls -l
```

The third print statement first interpolates the string, and then passes the result to the system. In Unix, "ls -l" produces a full directory listing, so our output might look something like:

```
total 50448
drwxr-xr-x    2 cjamison user     66 May 21 13:12 Desktop
drwxr-xr-x    2 cjamison user     44 Jun 18 22:41 admin
drwx------    2 cjamison user      9 May 22 12:44 autosave
drwxr-xr-x    3 cjamison user     24 Jun 18 22:39 courses
drwxr-xr-x    2 cjamison user     27 May 21 13:12 dumpster
drwx------    2 cjamison user      9 May 21 13:30 nsmail
drwxr-xr-x    3 cjamison user     28 May 22 10:12 projects
drwxr-xr-x    2 cjamison user   4096 May 22 10:15 ted_tmp
drwxr-xr-x    2 cjamison user     74 May 22 10:15 traces
```

2.5 Variable Definition

The act of creating a variable name is separate from the creation of the value. Until a specific value has been stored in the variable, the variable has a special value called 'undef' (short for undefined). The undef value is different from zero or the empty string, which are specific values in their own right (a variable might have a zero value because of a mathematical operation, which is very different than if it had never had a value put into it).

The defined() function takes a scalar variable and tests to see if the value is anything other than 'undef'. If it is, the function returns a true value, otherwise it returns a false value. The defined() function is usually used in conjunction with an if clause, which we will explore in Chapter 4.

Occasionally we might need to force a value to go away. To accomplish this task we use the undef() function, which given a particular variable name places the 'undef' value into it. Again, because 'undef' is a different value, this is different than simply assigning zero to the variable:

```
$var = 1;
defined($var); ## returns a TRUE value
$var = 0;
defined($var); ## returns a TRUE value
undef($var);
defined($var); ## returns a FALSE value
```

2.6 Special Variables

Perl has many predefined special variables that contain default values designed to make life easier for programmers. Most special variables are a combination of punctuation marks and obscure characters, and a programmer following the good coding practice of creating meaning variable names will never accidentally run into them. But, because all Perl variables can be reassigned, you won't get an error message if you accidentally tromp upon one. And because many of the special variables refer to arcane bits of the Perl language that many people don't ever use, debugging the horrible errors that occur from accidentally redefining one of the special variables is often a difficult job. Therefore, it does pay to be aware of the special variables just in case. Table 2.4 lists several that we will use in the coming chapters. For a complete listing see *Programming Perl, 3*rd *Ed.,* by Wall et al.

Chapter Summary

- A variable is a name for a data structure (a place to store data).
- Scalar variable names are prefixed with the $ character.
- Array variable names are prefixed with the @ character.
- Hash variable names are prefixed with the % character.
- Scalars are either numbers or character strings.
- Data type conversion is automatic.

Table 2.4 Special variables

Variable	Function
$_	default input and regexp search space
$/ and $\	input and output record separator
$,	output field separator
@ARGV	array with the command line arguments for the current script

- Operators are used to manipulate scalar variables.

- Variable interpolation occurs in strings surrounded by double quotes, but does not occur in strings surrounded by single quotes.

- The \ character is a backslash escape that protects a character from interpolation.

For More Information

```
perldoc perlsyn
perldoc perldata
```

Exercises

1. Which of the following are valid Perl variables? Explain what is wrong with the invalid variable names.

    ```
    $foo
    $foo bar
    $foo_bar
    $foo%bar
    $one_dark_and_stormy_night
    $101_dalmations
    ```

2. Which of the following scalar values are strings, and which are numbers?

    ```
    2
    A2
    2.3
    #2
    "2"
    '2'
    ```

3. What is the value of $i after each step of the following script?

    ```
    $i = 1;
    $i++;
    $i *= $i;
    $i .= $i;
    $i = $i/11;
    $i = $i . "score and" . $i + 3;
    ```

4. Explain the concept of interpolation.

5. If $a = 1 and $b = 2, what is the type and value of the scalar stored in $c after each of the following statements?

    ```
    $c = $a + $b;
    $c = $a / $b;
    $c = "$a + $b";
    $c = "$a + $b";
    ```

Programming Challenges

1. Create a script that tests your answers for Exercise 3. Try to explain any discrepancies between your answers and Perl's answers.

2. Write a script that calculates the slope and y intercept of the line determined by the two points (3, 4) and (15, 8). Print the line equation in the familiar form of "y = mx + b".

3. Create a script that tests your answers for Exercise 5. Try and explain any discrepancies between your answers and Perl's answers.

Chapter 3

Arrays and Hashes

Scalar values often are insufficient to deal with the data we use every day. For example, suppose we wanted to write a program that dealt with all the mapped genes on human chromosome 7, keeping track of the gene names and the sequence. With what we know so far, it would seem a simple task to create a variable named with the gene name (a safe proposition, inasmuch as the gene names on chromosome 7 are likely to be unique) and set the contents of that variable to a string showing the sequence:

```
$CFTR = 'aaaaaaaaaaa...';
```

The problem with this simple approach is that there are more than 550 mapped genes on chromosome 7, so we would have to create 550 variables: one for each gene. Clearly, that would become unwieldy. Simply initializing the variables would take a huge amount of space, and if we wanted to do something to each gene, we would have to write the same statement 550 times, changing only the variable name for the gene.

Fortunately, one of the philosophies of Perl is that laziness is a virtue. Two special types of variables exist to help manage long lists of items. Arrays and hashes make life easier, and are indispensable tools for the Perl programmer.

3.1 Arrays

A list is a simple concept. It is an ordered set of values. So if we wrote down all the mapped chromosome 7 genes starting from 7p22 and continuing on through

Perl Programming for Biologists,   D. Curtis Jamison
ISBN 0-471-43059-5   Copyright © 2003 Wiley-Liss, Inc.

7q36, we'd have an ordered list. To make life simple, let's concentrate on 7q31.2 and list the five mapped genes in order: CAPZA2, TFEC, CFTR, LOC51691, and LOC56311. In fact, the list we just wrote is almost the perfect definition of a Perl list. All we have to do is indicate the string boundaries, add parentheses, and lose the English grammar:

```
('CAPZA2', 'TFEC', 'CFTR', 'LOC51691', 'LOC56311')
```

The exact definition of a Perl list is a set of comma separated values enclosed in parentheses.

You can store a list in a special variable called an array. Array variable names are prefixed with an "@" symbol and follow the same rules as scalar variable names. Arrays can be created by assigning a list to an array variable:

```
@genes = ('CAPZA2', 'TFEC', 'CFTR', 'LOC51691', 'LOC56311');
```

The above line creates a nice little basket called @genes that we can use to carry around any number of gene names. Better, the values remain sorted and in order, so if we want to pull out the fourth gene, all we have to do is ask.

First though, let's look at the basket more closely. Figure 3.1 shows a picture of what that basket might look like. The first thing to note is that there is a unique numbered slot for each gene. The numbering keeps the items in the array in order. The second and most critical thing to note is that the first slot is numbered with a zero. The reason for this is historical, but the thing to remember is that real programmers count from zero.

We can access a value in the array by using the slot number as an index. Simply put the index number of the slot you want into square brackets, and append that to the end of the variable name (this process is called indexing into the array). Of course, now the variable is referring to a scalar value, so you have to use the $ symbol in front of the variable name, rather than the @ symbol:

```
print $genes[3];  # prints out LOC51691
```

Because each slot contains a scalar value, that means we can use each slot just like a scalar, and we can do anything to that slot that we can do with any other scalar. We can send it to the print function, or we can assign a new value to it. We can even use it in calculations.

One of the best things about Perl arrays is that they are dynamic: Slots are created on the fly. So, instead of creating the array with a single list, we can simply assign values into the proper slots and Perl takes care of creating the

0	CAPZA2
1	TFEC
2	CFTR
3	LOC51691
4	LOC56311

Figure 3.1   An array holding gene names

array. Thus

```
@genes = ('CAPZA2', 'TFEC', 'CFTR', 'LOC51691', 'LOC56311');
```

and

```
$genes[0] = 'CAPZA2';
$genes[1] = 'TFEC';
$genes[2] = 'CFTR';
$genes[3] = 'LOC51691';
$genes[4] = 'LOC56311';
```

both create an identical array. Even better, Perl doesn't care what order we fill the slots, so

```
$genes[0] = 'CAPZA2';
$genes[2] = 'CFTR';
$genes[3] = 'LOC51691';
$genes[4] = 'LOC56311';
$genes[1] = 'TFEC';
```

also creates an identical array. All three example produce an array that looks exactly like the picture in Figure 3.1.

In Perl, lists and arrays are almost interchangeable. Not only can we assign a list directly into an array, we can also assign an array back to a list of variables. In the latter operation, the first variable gets the value of the first slot, the second gets the second, and so on, until Perl runs out of either array slots or list variables. Thus

```
($a, $b, $c) = @genes;
```

sets $a, $b and $c to 'CAPZA2', 'TFEC', and 'CFTR', respectively, and ignores the rest of the entries in the array. Similarly,

```
($a, $b, $c, $d, $e, $f, $g) = @genes;
```

sets the values of the first five variables to the corresponding values in the array, and leaves $f and $g empty.

One tricky point to remember when dealing with lists is that Perl flattens lists when it interpolates them. So if you have a list within a list, or a list of arrays, the lists and arrays inside are treated as if each item was listed separately. Thus the list

```
('A', @genes, 'B')
```

and the list

```
('A', 'CAPZA2', 'TFEC', 'CFTR', 'LOC51691', 'LOC56311', 'B')
```

are identical. The trap novice Perl users sometimes fall into is trying to assign two lists into two arrays with a shortcut:

```
(@genes, @seqs) = (('TFEC', 'CTRF'),
                   ('atggctag', 'atagactaga'));
```

doesn't work like one might hope, assigning the gene names in the first list into @genes and the sequences in the second list into @seqs. Instead, even though the parentheses match up and it looks like it should work, the list on the right is flattened into a single list, and assigned into the @genes array, while the @seqs array remains empty.

3.3   Array Manipulation

3.3.1   Push and Pop, Shift and Unshift

When working with an array, we often don't know all the elements we want to store in the array ahead of time. Again, this is easy to deal with because Perl has dynamic arrays. We can add items to the end of the array with the push() function, and to the front of the array with the shift() function. The functions are very straightforward:

```
push(ARRAY, LIST)
unshift(ARRAY, LIST)
```

The push() function takes whatever items are in the list and appends them to the array, increasing the size of the array. So if we wanted to add the first five mapped genes in 7q31.31 we'd say

```
push(@genes, 'KCND2', 'NET-2', 'ING3','FLJ21986', 'WNT16');
```

and we'd get an array that looks like the one shown in Figure 3.2.

The unshift() function works in a similar way, but instead of appending the list, it inserts the list at the front of the array, shifting the existing entries over as many slots as needed. So, if we wanted to go the other direction and add the genes in 7q31.1 to the original @genes array, we would say

```
unshift(@genes, 'GPR85','DKFZP586B2022','CAV2','CAV1');
```

and we would have the array shown in Figure 3.3. Note that the indices have adjusted themselves, and CAPZA2 is now at index 4 rather than 0. This is a

0	CAPZA2
1	TFEC
2	CFTR
3	LOC51691
4	LOC56311
5	KCND2
6	NET-2
7	ING3
8	FLJ21986
9	WNT16

Figure 3.2   The array after values have been pushed onto it

0	GPR85
1	DKFZP586B2022
2	CAV2
3	CAV1
4	CAPZA2
5	TFEC
6	CFTR
7	LOC51691
8	LOC56311

Figure 3.3   New values shifted into the array from Figure 3.1.

0	TFEC
1	CFTR
2	LOC51691
3	LOC56311

Figure 3.4   The shifted array

feature of all array functions that insert or delete items at the front or middle of the array, and it guarantees that the order of the items in the list always remains the same.

Perl also has functions for removing items from the array. The pop() function removes the last item from the list, shortening it by one, and the shift() function removes the first item from the list, moving all entries over before shortening it by one. So, going back to the original array shown in Figure 3.1, we note that the CAPZA2 gene is actually not in 7q31.2, so we can shift it out of the array

```
shift(@genes);
```

and end up with the array shown in Figure 3.4.

Obviously, the push(), pop(), shift(), and unshift() functions make a rather awkward method of maintaining a list. The real power of these functions is that they return a value, which can be assigned to another variable. The value returned is the scalar that was in the slot that was popped or unshifted. So if we instead wrote

```
$first_gene = shift(@genes);
```

the @genes array still looks like Figure 3.4, while the $first_gene variable contains the string 'CAPZA2'. We can make use of these functions to chew through arrays of indeterminate length.

3.3.2   Splice

The most useful function for dealing with an array is the splice() function. The splice() function is the workhorse function for maintaining the entries in an array. Elements can be added and removed from the list, with the added advantage that the insertion or deletion can take place anywhere with the array, so if we want to remove a gene from the middle of our gene list we can do so quickly and easily.

Like many Perl functions, the splice() function has several incarnations and can be used in multiple ways to work with entries at both ends and in the middle of the array. The basic function looks like

```
splice(ARRAY, OFFSET, LENGTH, LIST)
```

The splice function takes an ARRAY, moves to the OFFSET slot, removes LENGTH entries, and replaces them with the entries from the LIST. The LENGTH and LIST are optional parameters, and the presence or absence of these two parameters determines the behavior of splice.

Let's examine the full behavior first. In our gene list, we can replace the entries for TFEC and CFTR with entries for four other genes:

```
splice(@genes, 1, 2, 'PAR3', 'NRP1', 'FLJ13031', 'EPC1');
```

Figure 3.5 illustrates the change in our array, which looks like a chromosomal translocation. The two genes from chromosome 7 are pushed out of the array, and the four new genes from chromosome 10 are put into their place. Note that the replaced genes aren't simply discarded, they are returned as an array we can capture and use later. This form of splice also works well if we want to insert some entries without deleting any first. We simply set the LENGTH to 0:

```
splice(@genes, 1, 0, 'PAR3', 'NRP1', 'FLJ13031', 'EPC1');
```

and we have the four chromosome 10 genes inserted in front of the gene in slot 1 while deleting zero existing, as shown in Figure 3.6.

If we leave out the replacement list from the arguments, we can delete entries from the array without adding any new items. In essence, we are giving the splice function a zero-length list of items to replace our specified items:

```
splice(@genes, 1, 2);
```

removes TFEC and CFTR from our original chromosome 7 array as shown in Figure 3.7.

Finally, splice can be used to truncate the array by leaving out both the length and the replacement list. When you do this, Perl assumes the length to delete is

0	CAPZA2
1	PAR3
2	NRP1
3	FLJ13031
4	EPC1
5	LOC51691
6	LOC56311

Figure 3.5 Using splice() to create a translocation

0	CAPZA2
1	PAR3
2	NRP1
3	FLJ13031
4	EPC1
5	TFEC
6	CFTR
7	LOC51691
8	LOC56311

Figure 3.6   Using splice to create an insertion

0	CAPZA2
1	LOC51691
2	LOC56311

Figure 3.7   Using splice to create a deletion

from the offset to the end of the array. Perhaps not the friendliest assumption, but that's the way it works, so

```
splice(@genes, 1);
```

replaces everything from the number one slot on with a zero-length list.

3.3.3   Other Useful Array Functions

Splice takes care of most of the things you need to do to manage arrays. But there are a couple other tasks that are so common with arrays that Perl has some built-in functions that save programmers time and make their programs run more efficiently. First, the reverse() function takes and array and returns an array in opposite order:

```
@inverse = reverse(@genes);
```

which produces the array in Figure 3.8.

The second common task is to sort an array. The sort() function has two forms. The first form takes an array and sorts it in standard string comparison order:

```
@alpha_list = sort(@genes);
```

0	LOC56311
1	LOC51691
2	CFTR
3	TFEC
4	CAPZA2

Figure 3.8   A reversed array

0	CAPZA2
1	CFTR
2	LOC51691
3	LOC56311
4	TFEC

Figure 3.9 A sorted array

which produces an array sorted in alphabetical order as shown in Figure 3.9. Again, note that each entry is now associated with a different index, reflecting the fact that we've altered the order.

Sometimes we don't want to sort strictly alphabetically. For example, maybe we'd like to sort a list of oligos based upon the length of the sequence. Thus, the second form of the sort function takes a subroutine as an argument, allowing the programmer to create a custom sorting algorithm. Sorting subroutines are covered in depth in Chapter 5.

3.3.4   List and Scalar Context

Perl defines two contexts for all variables to be interpolated under: scalar context and list context. Basically, this means that if Perl expects a list in a certain situation it treats whatever it is given in that situation like a list, and a scalar variable becomes a list with one element. Similarly, when an array is used in a scalar context, it behaves differently. Exactly how it behaves depends on the situation. For example, in most languages

```
$n = @genes;
```

would produce an error because you were attempting to assign an array to a scalar. But Perl is a bit smarter than the average language, and when an array is used in a scalar context, Perl assumes you want the count of items in the array. So, in a Perl program, the above statement would cause $n to have the value of 5.

Similarly, when you give the print function an array, Perl recognizes that you probably want to print the contents of each slot of the array, so the statement

```
print @genes;
```

produces the output

```
CAPZA2TFECCFTRLOC51691LOC56311
```

In this case, however, we'd like to impose a little bit of grammar and structure to make the line readable. We can do that a couple ways. First, we can simply put the entire string into double quotes. When Perl interpolates an array, it realizes that you probably want a string representation, so it separates each element with spaces:

```
print "@genes \n";
```

produces

```
CAPZA2 TFEC CFTR LOC51691 LOC56311
```

We can provide even more structure using the join() function, which takes a list and returns a string, with each element of the list separated by a user-specified string. The function looks like

```
join(STRING, LIST)
```

where STRING is the value used to separate each element of the LIST. So, to separate each element of our list with a comma and a space, we'd write a line like

```
print join(', ', (@genes, "\n"));
```

which would produce

```
CAPZA2, TFEC, CFTR, LOC51691, LOC56311,
```

Note that we created a list of our array and the "\n" character. Remember that when used in a list, the array gets flattened into the rest of the list. Therefore, when we joined the list, the "\n" got joined in at the end, giving the extra comma at the end of the list.

To avoid getting the extra comma, we need to first note the arguments to the join function look a lot like a list themselves. In fact, when arguments are passed to a function or a subroutine, they are passed as a list. If we omit the parentheses surrounding the join function, the function works fine because the arguments are interpreted in the list context:

```
$string1 = join(',', (@genes, "\n"));
$string2 = join ",", @genes, "\n";
print $string1;
print $string2;
```

produces two identical output lines.

Similarly, the print function we have been using to print out strings takes a list of arguments. Until now, we have been providing a list one item long, and omitting the redundant parentheses. But if we were to supply a list, the print function would write out each item in the list concatenated together, just like it did with the @gene array. So with a little judicious editing of the parentheses, we can create a print statement with two scalars in the argument list: a string created by the join function, and a new line character:

```
print join(',',(@genes)), "\n";
```

The join function concatenates the @genes array into a comma-separated string, and then print statement prints the string concatenated with the new-line character, getting rid of the annoying extra comma. Note that in this case the parentheses around the argument list for the join function are required to tell the join function where its list ends.

Occasionally though, the context you're using the array in prevents you from doing exactly what you want to do. For example, what if we wanted to print out the number of elements in an array? We know that putting a bare array into a print statement gets us the elements printed out, as does putting the array into double quotes. And, of course, putting the array into single quotes simply prints out the variable name. So none of the three statements

```
print 'array has', @genes, 'elements', "\n";
print "array has @genes elements\n";
print 'array has @genes elements\n';
```

gets us the printout we desire, because we never get @genes into a scalar context. So one way to get the information would be to take an extra line and force the issue:

```
$gene_count = @array;
print "array has $gene_count elements\n";
```

which outputs

```
array has 5 elements
```

Another way would be to use the scalar() function, which forces an expression to be interpolated in a scalar context. So we could have written

```
print 'array has', scalar(@genes), 'elements', "\n";
```

and gotten the same result by forcing the @genes array to be interpreted in the scalar context.

One of the most beautiful aspects of Perl is that there are many ways of doing things, and there is no single "right answer" when approaching a problem. We have also seen that most of the common issues programmers face have already been anticipated. Thus, it should come as no surprise that there is another, simpler way to get the count of an array.

We always know the beginning index of an array, because under normal conditions all arrays begin at 0. But it is often quite useful to know the final index of an array, perhaps to look at the final value without removing it using pop(). So a special array syntax exists to get the last index: replace the @ symbol with $# in the variable name and you access a predefined variable that came into existence along with your array. The $# variable contains the scalar value of the final index.

So $#genes contains the value 4, which is the final index in the array. Adding 1 to the $# value gives a count of how many slots are in the array. Thus, we can write our code to be a little more compact:

```
print 'array has ', $#genes+1, 'elements', "\n";
```

which outputs the same answer as the other methods:

```
array has 5 elements
```

3.4 Hashes

Now that we know about arrays, let's revisit the original problem. Remember we have a list of gene names and their associated sequences, and we want to store them in our Perl program. We could create one array for gene names and a second array for the sequences:

```
$genes[0] = 'CAPZA2';
$seqs[0] = 'ATGTGGTG...'; #sequence for CAPZA2
$genes[1] = 'TFEC';
$seqs[1] = 'ATGTGGTG...'; #sequence for TFEC
$genes[2] = 'CFTR';
$seqs[2] = 'ATGTGGTG...'; #sequence for CFTR
$genes[3] = 'LOC51691';
$seqs[3] = 'ATGTGGTG...'; #sequence for LOC51691
$genes[4] = 'LOC56311';
$seqs[4] = 'ATGTGGTG...'; #sequence for LOC56311
```

With parallel arrays, we can now get the sequence associated with a gene name simply by using the same index to access both arrays. For example, if we wanted to print a sequence in something approximating a FASTA file format[2] (see Appendix B) we could write code like:

```
print "> $genes[0] \n$seqs[0]\n";
```

This technique works well as long as we're extremely careful to keep the two arrays in register. If we apply the pop() function to @genes, we must apply the pop() function to @seqs. If we don't, then suddenly we have more sequences than names. Worse, if we were to accidentally pop() one array and shift() another, the remaining sequences would no longer match to the right gene names.

Fortunately, there is a data structure implemented in Perl that takes care of a lot of these problems. A hash is a special kind of array that uses strings for naming the array slots rather than numbers. The string that names a slot is called the key, and the item in the slot is called the value. Together, these two entities make up a key-value pair, and a hash is a structure that associates the key and value together for storage and later retrieval.

Hashes are named by prefixing the variable name with the % symbol. Otherwise, the normal naming conventions apply. Hashes can be initialized by a list, similar to the list used for an ordinary array, but in this case the list is arranged into alternating key-value pairs:

```
%sequences = ( 'CAPZA2', 'ATGTGGTG...',
               'TFEC', 'ATGTGGTG...',
               'CFTR','ATGTGGTG...',
               'LOC51691', 'ATGTGGTG...',
               'LOC56311', 'ATGTGGTG...');
```

---

[2]This only approximates the FASTA file format, since the entire sequence is printed on a single line.

Figure 3.10   An hash for sequences

This function produces a hash that looks something like the one shown in Figure 3.10.

Alternately, instead of using a list we can use the hash assignment notation,[3] which is an = sign followed by the > sign. Thus we can rewrite our function as

```
%sequences = (CAPZA2 =>'ATGTGGTG...',
                TFEC =>'ATGTGGTG...',
                CFTR =>'ATGTGGTG...',
                LOC51691 =>'ATGTGGTG...',
                LOC56311 =>'ATGTGGTG...');
```

Notice that we removed the quotes around the keys. When we use the => notation, Perl assumes that the key is going to be a string.

Indexing into the hash is done in a method similar to indexing into a regular array, except that we use the curly braces { and } instead of brackets, and you put a string in as the reference. So to print the sequence for CFTR, we would write

```
print $sequences{'CFTR'};
```

and to make a pseudo-Fasta output like we did above, we would write

```
print "> CFTR \n$sequences{'CFTR'}\n";
```

Hashes get their name because the keys are stored in a data structure called a hash table. Hash table lookups are very fast, so the performance of getting things in and out of hashes is very good. However, storing the keys in a hash table means that the key-value pairs are no longer in the same order as we put them into the hash. Thus hashes are unordered, which is an important fact to remember when we try and get values back out, because we will probably want to impose some sort of order.

3.5   Maintaining a Hash

Adding new key-value pairs to a hash is simple. Like a normal array, an entry in a hash can be created by assigning a value into an indexed slot. So, we could have created %sequences by writing:

---

[3]Note that this is a little white lie: there really isn't a hash assignment notation. The => is actually a synonym for the comma. So be forewarned, because you may see some really weird code that says a =>b =>c or something like that. However, it is usually easier to think of it as the hash assignment notation.

```
$sequences{'CAPZA2'} = 'ATGTGGTG...';
$sequences{'TFEC'} = 'ATGTGGTG...';
$sequences{'CFTR'} = 'ATGTGGTG...';
$sequences{'LOC51691'} = 'ATGTGGTG...';
$sequences{'LOC56311'} = 'ATGTGGTG...';
```

Deleting entries is a little more tricky. If we simply assign a zero to a slot, the key still exists (as it should – often we know a gene name without knowing the sequence). Similarly, if we simply use the undef() function the key is still present:

```
undef($sequences{'TFEC'});
```

leaves us a hash that looks like Figure 3.11, with the "TFEC" key still present in the hash.

But if we want to remove the entry completely so that no trace of the TFEC gene remains, we have to do a little more. Perl provides the delete() function to take care of both the key and value. The delete function removes a variable name from the namespace, completely expunging it. Obviously, this is a function to be careful with, but

```
delete($sequences{'TFEC'});
```

has the desired effect and makes our hash look like Figure 3.12.

Perl also provides some functions specifically for working with hashes. The keys() function returns a list of all the keys in the given hash. So, in the case of the %sequences array, we would get a list of all the gene names. Similarly, the values() function returns a list of the values, which would be the actual sequences in %sequences. The lists returned from these functions can be used in a regular array. For example:

```
@gene_names = sort(keys(%sequences));
```

creates an alphabetical list of all the gene names we used as keys, and stores the list in the @gene_names array.

CAPZA2	ATGTGGTG
TFEC	
CFTR	ATGTGGTG
LOC51691	ATGTGGTG
LOC56311	ATGTGGTG

Figure 3.11 A null value associated with the TFEC key

CAPZA2	ATGTGGTG
CFTR	ATGTGGTG
LOC51691	ATGTGGTG
LOC56311	ATGTGGTG

Figure 3.12 The TFEC key expunged by delete()

Finally, the each() function gives back a two-element list that consists of the key-value pair for the next element of a hash. When coupled with a while loop, the each function allows you to iterate over all the key-values pairs in the hash. Typically, people use an assignment from the each() function to a two variable list:

```
($key, $value) = each(%sequences)
```

We'll see this in a real example in Chapter 4.

Chapter Summary

- An array is the Perl data type that contains lists.

- Arrays are indexed by numbers beginning from 0.

- Array values are accessed by using the index.

- Arrays are manipulated with the push(), pop(), shift(), unshift(), and splice() functions.

- Lists can be assigned to arrays, and an array can be assigned to a list of scalar variables.

- Hashes (hashes) are indexed by strings rather than numbers.

- Hash values are accessed by the index string.

For More Information

```
perldoc perldata
```

Exercises

1. For the following array declaration

```
@myArray = ('A', 'B', 'C', 'D', 'E');
```

what is the value of the following expressions?

```
$#myArray
length(@myArray)
$myArray[1]
```

2. What is the difference between a list and an array?

3. A queue is a special type of list that keeps the elements in order and adds or removes elements only from the ends of the list. Queues can be simulated with Perl arrays and judicious use of the push, pop, shift, and unshift operators. Explain which operators you would you to make a FIFO

queue ("first-in, first-out," like the line at the grocery store checkout), and which operators you would use to create a LIFO queue ("last-in, first-out," like a Pez dispenser).

4. Which of the following are valid keys for a hash?

   ```
   'CAPZ'
   '12'
   '$key'
   $key
   ```

5. Hash keys need to be unique. In the following data pairs, indicate which should be the key and which should be the value.

a. Gene Name	b. Genetic Distance
a. Species	b. Ecosystem
a. Plate well	b. Gene Name
a. Accession	b. Gene Name
a. Sequence	b. Accession

Programming Challenge

1. Write a Perl statement that counts the number of entries in a hash.

Chapter 4

Control Structures

Thus far, we have seen how to create scalar, array, and hash variables. Now we need to perform a task with these variables. To do so, we need to learn about the control structures available in Perl.

A control structure is a little bit like a function, in that it takes an argument and does something with it. However, rather than performing a transformation on the argument, a control structure evaluates the argument for truth and then executes the statements following depending on whether the argument evaluates to true or false. Which brings up the age-old question: what is truth?

For programmers, truth is easier to define in terms of what is not truth. In Perl, there is a short, specific list of false values:

- zero,

- undef,

- an empty string, and

- and empty list.

Any expression that returns a value not in the list is true.

So, the argument for a control structure is some sort of Perl statement that can be evaluated. Many Perl functions return a value that can be used as the argument for a control structure: we saw this in the use of the defined() function in Chapter 2, which returns a false value if the variable is 'undef'. In fact, defined() actually returns the undef value. Another way to build an expression that returns a true or false value is to use the built-in Perl comparison operators.

Perl Programming for Biologists, D. Curtis Jamison
ISBN 0-471-43059-5 Copyright © 2003 Wiley-Liss, Inc.

4.1   Comparisons

Everyone is familiar with comparison operators. These are the symbols we used in algebra to indicate whether numbers were greater than or less than another. When we use these in programming, the value on the left is compared to the value on the right, and a number is returned, either 1 if the assertion is true, or undef if the assertion is false. Table 4.1 lists the operators available in Perl.

The first thing to note is that the numeric comparison operators look a little different than we remember. Perl doesn't use the fancy fonts that text editors do, so symbols like $\neq$, $\geq$, and $\leq$ don't exist, and we have to use two-symbol approximations for them. Second, notice that the numeric comparison for equality is two = symbols. This is because Perl uses the single = symbol as the assignment operator. The double==symbol keeps straight the difference between assignments and comparisons. Finally, the signed result equality comparison <=> is a useful if somewhat tricky operator. This operator compares two values, but with a twist. If the two items being compared are equal it returns false, whereas if the two are not equal the operator returns a 1 if the right item is larger and a −1 if the left item is larger. Remember that both 1 and −1 qualify as truth for Perl, and the sign simply indicates the direction the truth is pointing.

The string comparison operators parallel the numeric operators, but instead of using symbols they use short mnemonics. This is because we need to tell Perl whether we are using the value as a number or as a string, because Perl will autoconvert between the two for us, often with unexpected results. For example, look at what happens when we confuse the numeric signed equality operator with the string signed equality operator:

```
$a = 100;
$b = 30;
$c = $a <=> $b;  # $c contains a 1
$d = $a cmp $b;  # $d contains a -1
```

The value stored in $c is quite understandable: because 100 is greater than 30, the value returned is a positive 1. On the other hand, when we compare the

Table 4.1   Perl comparison operators

Numeric Comparison	String Comparison	Question
$a = = $b	$a eq $b	Is $a equal to $b?
$a ! = $b	$a ne $b	Is $a not equal to $b?
$a > $b	$a gt $b	Is $a greater than $b?
$a > = $b	$a ge $b	Is $a greater than or equal to $b?
$a < $b	$a lt $b	Is $a less than $b?
$a < = $b	$a le $b	Is $a less than or equal to $b?
$a <=> $b	$a cmp $b	Is $a not equal to $b? (with signed result)

values as strings, we get the opposite result indicating that "100" is less than "30". This is due to the special way that Perl works string comparisons.

When Perl compares two strings, it takes the leftmost character of each string and compares them. If the two characters are identical, it takes the next two to the right and compares them, and so on, until it finds a pair of characters that are not identical. If it reaches the end of both strings without finding any different characters, then the two string are identical and therefore are equal.

However, as soon as it finds a pair of characters that are different, the two strings are no longer equal. The metric Perl uses is the character's position in the character table. The character table is an ordered list of all possible characters, rather much like an array. Each character in the list has an index, and to compare two characters, Perl simply does a numeric comparison of their indices. Characters further into the table are considered to be greater than characters earlier in the table. Thus 'a' is less than 'z', and 'a' is less than 'A' (Perl is case-sensitive). So in our example above, when 100 and 30 were compared as strings, Perl started at the first letter and found that '1' is less than '3' so therefore the signed equality operator returned a −1.

A special case in string comparisons occurs when two strings are identical at all positions but one string is longer than another, like "cow" and "cows". By definition, the longer string is considered to be greater. So

```
"cow" cmp "cows"
```

returns a −1.

4.2   Choices

4.2.1   If

The most fundamental control structure is the if statement. The if statement is used to protect a block of code that only needs to be executed if a prior condition is (or isn't) met. The general format for an if statement is

```
if (expression) { code block }
```

The expression in parentheses is the condition we are testing. After the conditional expression is a code block. A code block is a set of instruction statements grouped together by curly braces. The control statement executes the code block if the conditional is true.

An if statement is useful to check a variable to make sure it is within reasonable bounds:

```
if ($gene_count > $max_genes) {
    die "You have too many genes!\n";
}
```

This piece of code checks for an error condition and invokes the die() function, which prints out an error statement and exits the program. Error checking can be very important to avoid asking the program to divide by zero or work on a value that doesn't exist, tasks that usually result in Perl giving an error statement and quitting. Typically, this occurs after an operation when you want to make sure of the results. For example, if we invoke pop() on an empty array the return value is undef, and we can check that:

```
$value = pop(@empty_array);
if (! $value) {
  die "Popped an empty array\n";
}
```

This chunk of code, like the one before it, will exit the program with an appropriate error message if there was nothing in the array. The exclamation point (often pronounced "not") is the Boolean negate, and inverses the result. So, if $value is false, the negation is true.

Thus far, we have used the if statement to deal with single choice errors where we have aborted the entire program when the error exists. More commonly, we use the if statement to encapsulate a chunk of code that applies to a specific condition, and we wish to do a calculation. For example, we might want to round a map position to two decimal points before continuing with our program:

```
$truncate = int($position * 100) / 100;
if ($position - $truncate >= .005) {
  $truncate += .01;
}
$position = $truncate;
```

The first line shifts the decimal point two positions to the right, uses the int() function to turn the value from a floating point into an integer (effectively chopping off everything after the decimal), then shifts the decimal point back two places to the left by dividing by 100. This leaves a floating point value that has been truncated after the second decimal point. The if statement then checks to see if the third digit after the decimal point is 5 or higher, and rounds the truncated number upwards if true. The last statement then puts the rounded value back into the $position variable.

Note that after evaluating an if statement, Perl will either execute or skip the controlled code block, then will pick up with the very next statement. Control structures like the if statement are sometimes called branch points, because they create an alternative code branch to follow.

4.2.2 Boolean Operators

Sometimes more than one condition factors into a decision. For example, suppose we have some hashes containing information about genes on our map: %genetic contains genetic map positions and %physical contains the physical map position of the start code. Each array is indexed by the gene name. Now we want to check and see if a particular gene has both a genetic and a physical map position. We could do this by nesting a pair of if statements:

```
$gene = 'CFTR';
if (defined($genetic{$gene})) {
  if (defined($physical{$gene})) {
    print "$gene is on both maps\n";
  }
}
```

First we check for a value in %genetic, and if true when then check for a value in %physical, and if true when then print a message. Although this method works, Perl provides a cleaner way to do this with Boolean logical operators. The Boolean AND operation is provided by the && operator, and the Boolean OR operator is provided by the ‖ operator. These operators tie together a pair of expressions and then combine their result. The AND operator returns true if the expressions on both sides evaluate to true, and the OR operator returns true if either side evaluates to true. Thus we can use a Boolean operator to rewrite our code using a single if statement:

```
$gene = 'CFTR';
if (defined($genetic{$gene}) && defined($physical{$gene})) {
  print "$gene is on both maps\n";
}
```

This expression is both cleaner and easier to understand. Plus, an added bonus is that it will execute faster. It takes a little time to set up a branch, so the fewer if statements the faster the code runs.

Any number of Boolean operators can be chained together. If we added a third hash to hold RH map data, we could check and see if the gene is on all three maps:

```
$gene = 'CFTR';
if (defined($genetic{$gene})
    && defined($physical{$gene})
    && defined($rh{$gene}) {
  print "$gene is on both maps\n";
}
```

Note that we took advantage of Perl's ability to ignore white space to make our expression a little more readable. Even though the expression is spread across several lines and several tabs, Perl read through the extraneous white space until it reached the closing parenthesis.

Like all operators, Boolean operators have a specific precedence, and fit into the general list of operators. The negate operator ! that we saw in the previous section has the highest precedence, followed by the && and the ‖ operators. There are also synonymous operators 'not', 'and', and 'or' which have an extremely low precedence.

4.2.3 Else

When making a choice, sometimes you have two different things you wish to do, depending upon the outcome of the conditional. Maybe we want also want to print a message when the gene is not on both maps. Again, we could use two if statements

```
$gene = 'CFTR';
if (defined($genetic{$gene})
      && defined($physical{$gene})) {
   print "$gene is on both maps\n";
}
if (! (defined($genetic{$gene})
      && defined($physical{$gene}))) {
   print "$gene is not on both maps\n";
}
```

but that looks a little repetitive. In fact, aside from having to set up a second branch, the program has to re-evaluate a statement and therefore this construction is rather wasteful of time. Because Perl programmers abhor wasting time, it is no surprise that there is a control structure for this common situation. The else statement follows an if statement, and provides an alternative block of code to perform when the if statement is false:

```
if (EXPR) {code block} else {code block}
```

So we can write our map-checking code as

```
$gene = 'CFTR';
if (defined($genetic{$gene}) && defined($physical{$gene})) {
   print "$gene is on both maps\n";
} else {
   print "$gene is not on both maps\n";
}
```

Perl evaluates the if conditional and either executes the block of code controlled by the if or the block of code controlled by the else, depending on the value of the condition. After executing one block or the other, Perl skips to the statement following the else block and continues on.

Perl also provides a control structure to use if there are multiple combinations of factors and more than two possible choices. The elsif is a hybrid of the else and the if statement. It gives an else to jump to if the proceeding condition was false, and a new if expression to evaluate to decide whether to execute the next block. Any number of elsifs can follow an if, and a string of elsif statements can be followed by an else to provide a default code block to execute:

```
if (EXPR) {code block} elsif (EXPR) {code block} else {code block}
```

Using this construct, we can check to see if our gene can be found on any combination of maps:

```
$gene = 'CFTR';
if (defined($genetic{$gene})
      && defined($physical{$gene})
      && defined($rh{$gene}) {
   print "$gene is on all maps\n";
```

```
  } elsif (defined($genetic{$gene})
          && defined($physical{$gene})) {
    print "$gene is on genetic and physical maps\n";
  } elsif (defined($genetic{$gene})
          && defined($rh{$gene})) {
    print "$gene is on genetic and RH maps\n";
  } elsif (defined($physical{$gene})
          && defined($physical{$gene})) {
    print "$gene is on physical and RH maps\n";
  } else {
    print "$gene is not on multiple maps\n";
  }
```

There are a couple of commonly used shortcuts that are used in Perl. First, it is fairly common to write an if conditional that is looking for a false value. We can either write a Boolean negator into the expression like we did before, or we can use the unless control structure. The unless is used exactly like an if, except the sense of the test is reversed:

```
if (! $value) {die "Popped an empty array\n";}
unless ($value) {die "Popped an empty array\n";}
```

These do exactly the same thing. Neither is particularly superior to the other, and deciding which one to use is often a stylistic choice designed to make reading a program easier.

The other shortcut involves the Boolean || operator. Perl is smart enough to recognize that it only needs to evaluate one side of the || at a time: If the first side is true then the entire statement is true, so Perl does not bother to evaluate the right side. Programmers take advantage of this short circuit and write lines of code that contain alternate statements on either side of the operator. This is usually used to monitor a Perl function or a subroutine that must return a true value. For example, almost every program that opens a file uses a line like:

```
open(FILE, "filename") || die "Couldn't open $file\n";
```

This statement is essentially a bare conditional expression. Perl first evaluates the left-hand side to see if it is true. If open succeeds in making the file listed available, it returns a true value and Perl then continues on without bothering to evaluate the rest of the conditional. However, if open fails and returns false, then Perl needs to check the right-hand side to see whether it is true, and when it evaluates the die function it exits the program. We'll see more about the open function in Chapter 7.

4.3 Loops

When most people figure out how an array works, one of the first obvious things they want to do with it is to apply a code block to every item in the array. We've already seen how to work with single entries, like printing out the sequence for a gene name, but suppose you wanted to print out the sequence for every gene? Either you would have to write a code block for each gene name, or you would have to write a generic code block and figure out a way to apply that code to every item in the array. Loops allow you to do that.

Every loop has three main parts: an entry condition that starts the loop, a code block that serves as the body of the loop, and an exit condition. The entry and exit conditions are important, and are related. Obviously, without a proper entry condition your program can never enter the loop, and without an exit condition your program will never exit the loop. A missing or misconceived exit condition leads to a state known as a continuous loop, where the program keeps going around and around forever. A classic example of an infinite loop is the shampoo algorithm:

```
Lather
Rinse
Repeat
```

Examine the loop carefully. If you interpret each line literally, you'll see that you will never actually finish, because the repeat function sends you back to the beginning every time.

There are two types of loops: determinate and indeterminate. Determinate loops carry their exit condition with them from the beginning, and repeat a code block an exact number of times. Indeterminate loops rely upon code within the body of the loop to alter the exit condition so the loop can exit.

4.3.1 For Loops

The most basic type of determinant loop is the for loop. This control structure has the syntax

```
for (ENTRY; TEST; MODIFICATION) {code block}
```

The ENTRY expression sets up the entry condition, and the TEST expression sets up the exit condition. The MODIFICATION expression tells Perl how to modify the entry condition. When Perl finds a for loop,

- it sets up the entry condition,
- examines the test condition,
- executes the code block if the test is true,
- modifies the test condition, and then
- goes back to the test.

Thus

```
for ($i = 0; $i < 5; $i++) {print "$i\n";}
```

prints out

```
0
1
2
3
4
```

The entry code was to set $i to 0, and the test said $i<5 was true, so Perl printed 0. Then $i was autoincremented to 1, tested to be less than five, and so on until the last iteration of the loop set autoincremented $i from 4 to 5, which caused the test to fail and the loop to exit. Note that if the test fails, the for loop exits immediately without performing the loop:

```
for($i = 10; $i < 5; $i++) {print "$i\n";}'
```

prints out nothing, because the entry condition fails the test and the loop exits without going into the body.

One cautionary note about the variable used to control the for loop: the variable joins the namespace of the program. So, after executing the for loop $i is defined and has the value it had when the loop exited. If we try to print the value of $i after the loop:

```
for($i = 0; $i < 5; $i++) {print "$i\n";}
print "$i\n";
```

we find the output from the code above would be

```
0
1
2
3
4
5
```

We can get around this problem by restricting the $i variable to the for loop using the my command:

```
for(my $i = 0; $i < 5; $i++) {print "$i\n";}
print "$i\n";
```

outputs

```
0
1
2
3
4
```

The $i inside the for loop is a temporary variable, which only has value inside the for loop, and outside the for loop it has an undef value (and so prints an empty string). Because the variable is a temporary variable, it can also save the value of a variable from getting crunched:

```
$i = 89;
for(my $i = 0; $i < 5; $i++) {print "$i\n";}
print "$i\n";
```

prints out

```
0
1
2
3
4
89
```

The my command has saved the value of the $i outside the loop. The my command affects the scope of the $i variable, a subject we will cover in more depth in Chapter 5.

For loops are very useful for iterating over the items in an array. For example, we can use a for loop to print out each value in the @genes array from Chapter 3. Remember there were five genes names in the array, so the for loop would look like:

```
for ($i = 0; $i < 5; $i++) {print $genes[$i], "\n";}
```

and would produce the output:

```
CAPZA2
TFEC
CFTR
LOC51691
LOC56311
```

(of course, we could have accomplished the same thing with

```
print join("\n", @genes);
```

but that's beside the point).

A slightly more general variant of this example is

```
for ($i = 0; $i <= $#genes; $i++) {print $genes[$i], "\n";}
```

This code variant produces the exact same output as before, but now we are testing to see if the value of $i is less than or equal to the last index in @genes. This allows us to print the contents of the array no matter how large the array is, even if we don't know the exact number of items. Note that even though we don't know how big the array really is, the for loop is still determinant because it will execute exactly $#genes times, and Perl knows what the value of $#genes is even if we don't.

4.3.2   Foreach Loops

In fact, the use of a for loop for iterating over each item in an array is so common, that Perl has a special shortcut for loop specifically for this task, the foreach loop:

```
foreach $VAR (@ARRAY) {code block}
```

The foreach loop takes each value in @ARRAY, places it into $VAR, and executes the code block. It exits when there are no more elements in the array. So we could write our code like so:

```
foreach $gene (@genes) {print "$gene\n";}
```

which is just as effective, and probably even more readable than the other variants.

Even better, the foreach loop in conjunction with the keys() function gives us an easy way to iterate over a hash. Remember that keys() gives back a list of the index values, so we could access each element of the %sequence hash from Chapter 3 and write out a FASTA-like sequence for every sequence:

```
foreach $key (keys(%sequences)) {
  print ">$key \n$sequences{$key}\n\n";
}
```

would produce

```
>CAPZA2
ATGTGGTG...

>TFEC
ATGTGGTG...

>CFTR
ATGTGGTG...

>LOC51691
ATGTGGTG...

>LOC56311
ATGTGGTG...
```

which is, essentially, a FASTA library (except that the sequences are printed out on a single line).

The foreach loop is also very useful for inverting a hash. Sometimes it is useful to extract data from a hash based upon the value rather than the key. For example, remember the %genetic array, which is keyed by the gene name and contains the genetic map position. Rather than asking what position is a gene at, we might want to know which genes are at a particular position. We could iterate across the array, checking to see if the current key is at the position we're interested in:

```
@genelist = ();
foreach $gene (keys(%genetic)) {
  if ($genetic{$gene} eq '7p32') {
    push(@genelist, $gene);
  }
}
print join(", ", @genelist, "\n");
```

Because there may be multiple genes at any particular genetic position, we capture the genes in a temporary array and then print out the array. Although this method works, the code would need to be run every time we wanted to ask this particular question, and we would have to run through the entire array multiple times. It would be better to be able to create the inverted array once, then we could query it multiple times much more quickly:

```
foreach $gene (keys(%genetic)) {
  $position = $genetic{$gene};
  if ($inv_genetic{$position}) {
    @tmp = ($inv_genetic{$position});
  } else {
    @tmp = ();
  }
  push(@tmp, $gene);
  $inv_genetic{$genetic{$gene}} = join(",", @tmp);
}
```

This code creates a second hash. The key for %inv_genetic is the position, which is the value in %genetic, and the value is a string that contains the gene names separated by commas (which looks a lot like a list, and in fact can be interpolated into one). So this foreach loop takes each gene name from the array returned by the keys function, then creates a temporary holding variable called $position. We then check to see whether we already created a string for that particular position. If we have, we interpolate the string into a temporary array, and if we haven't we create a blank temporary array. Then we push the gene name onto our array, and finally we turn the array back into a string using the join function, inserting the string into the inverted secondary array.

The new inverted array allows us to either query with a specific position, or we could iterate over the entire inverted array and print out the string of gene names by position:

```
foreach $pos (keys(%inv_genetic)) {
  print "$pos: $inv_genetic{$pos}\n";
}
```

which would produce a output that looked something like

```
7q10: gene1,gene5
7q11: gene7,gene3
7p32: gene8,gene2,gene4,gene6
```

4.4   Indeterminate Loops

4.4.1   While

Often we find a situation where neither we nor Perl know in advance how many times a loop will need to execute. For example, if we are reading lines from a file, we may not know exactly how many lines there are. This is where the while loop comes in handy. The while loop control structure looks like

```
while (TEST) {code block}
```

The while loop executes the code block as long as the TEST expression evaluates as true. A very simple example of a while loop is

```
$i = 0;
while ($i < 50) {
  print "$i\n";
  $i++;
}
```

The entry condition is set outside the loop. When entering the loop, Perl first evaluates the test expression, and then if true, executes the code block. Perl then checks the test again and decides whether to execute the block again or to exit the loop and continue on. In this example, the loop will print out the digits 0 through 49.

Now, we could have written the while loop as a determinate loop:

```
for ($i = 0; $i < 50; $i++) {
  print "$i\n";
}
```

Viewed this way, the three parts of the loop can be seen clearly: The entry condition of $i=0, the test of $i<50, and the modification of $i++. The major difference between the two versions is the layout. In the for loop, all three parts are integral to the control structure, but the while loop relies upon code before or within the code block. As it turns out, every determinate loop can be written as an indeterminate loop. For example,

```
for ($i = 0; $i <= $#genes; $i++) {print $genes[$i], "\n";}
```

can be rewritten as

```
$i = 0;
while ($i <= $#genes) {
  print $genes[$i], "\n";
  $i++;
}
```

and even a foreach loop for a hash

```
foreach $key (keys(%sequences)) {
  print "> $key \n$sequences{$key}\n\n";
}
```

can be written in a while loop (with the help of the each() function from Chapter 3):

```
while ((%key, $seq) = each(%sequences)) {
  print "> $key \n$seq\n\n";
}
```

which produces the exact same output.

So if we can write any for loop as a while loop, why do we need a for loop? It turns out the for loop is much more efficient for Perl to translate into machine language, and so for loops run a bit faster than while loops. But there are often cases where the while loop is unavoidable.

For example, let's look at the case of the %inv_genetic hash. Remember, this array is set up so that the keys are map positions and the values are a list of genes. From this array we output a report that listed map position and gene list. Now, suppose we wanted to write the report for the first 50 or so genes. That means we need to write out the lists while keeping track of how many gene names we've written. Because we don't know ahead of time how many gene names there are per line, we have to use a while loop:

```
$count = 0;
@indices = sort(keys(%inv_genetic));
$index = 0;
while ($count < 50) {
  print "$indices[$index]: $inv_genetic{$indices[$index]}\n";
  @tmp = ($inv_genetic{$indices[$index]});
  $count += $#tmp + 1;
  $index++;
}
```

First, we create the test variable $count and set it to 0. Then we make an array of the indices for %inv_genetics, sorting it so they will be in order, and we also create the $index variable, which we will use to keep our place in the array. Now we can start our while loop, setting the test condition to be 50 or fewer. We then print a line of our report. Next, we interpolate the gene name string into a temporary array so we can count how many gene names we just printed out and add them to our total in $count. Finally, we increment $index so we can get the next key.

4.4.2   Repeat Until

Because looping across a set of statements is a common task in Perl, a special loop control structure just for that purpose. The logic behind the repeat-until loop is similar to that of the while:

```
$count = 0;
@indices = sort(keys(%inv_genetic));
$index = 0;
repeat {
  print "$indices[$index]: $inv_genetic{$indices[$index]}\n";
  @tmp = ($inv_genetic{$indices[$index]});
  $count += $#tmp + 1;
  $index++;
} until ($count < 50);
```

performs the exact same task as the while loop. The difference between the loops is mainly cosmetic, with the code block up front and the conditional expression trailing. Some people prefer to use the repeat-until construct because it makes the code read more like English.

4.5   Loop Exits

One issue that is important in complex loops is the manner in which you handle errors. Sometimes a situation arises where continuing with the current code block is either unnecessary or undesirable. Perl provides a few functions that can be used to control loops from inside the code block.

4.5.1   Last

Often a situation arises where an error condition makes continuing in the loop will lead to grave problems. In some cases, you might wish to go ahead and exit the entire program using the die() function, but that is not always necessary (and certainly not particularly friendly). If you just want to get out of the loop and continue the program, the last() function will cause the loop to exit prematurely.

For example, in the previous while loop we forgot to make sure we actually had 50 gene names to iterate over. If we don't have 50 entries, the while loop will try to access slots even though $index is beyond the last index, and Perl will generate a series of undefined values. So, we can check and then exit the loop if we need to:

```
$count = 0;
@indices = sort(keys(%inv_genetic));
$index = 0;
while ($count < 50) {
  if ($index > $#indices) {last;}
  print "$indices[$index]: $inv_genetic{$indices[$index]}\n";
  @tmp = $inv_genetic{$indices[$index]};
  $count += $#tmp + 1;
  $index++;
}
```

The if statement checks to see whether the $index is greater than the last index in @indices, and if so the last() function immediately skips to the next statement after the loop.

4.5.2   Next and Continue

Other times, you might just want to skip a single iteration of a loop. In this case, the next function is used to advance to the next iteration of the loop. For example, if you only wanted to print out a FASTA file for gene names that started with the letter "c", you could write"

```
foreach $key (keys(%sequences)) {
  if (! ($key gt 'C' && $key lt 'D')) {next;}
  print "> $key \n$sequences{$key}\n\n";
}
```

In a for and foreach loop, the next operator automatically performs the modification of the loop condition. However, in a while loop the modification is usually internal to the code block (some test expressions are self-modifying, like the each() function). If the next statement is encountered before the modification to the loop control, then you've created an infinite loop:

```
$i = 1;
while ($i < 50) {
  if (! $i%2) {next;}
  print "$i\n";
  $i++;
}
```

which is an attempt to print out only the odd numbers from 1 to 50. But if you walk through the loop, you'll see that when $i = 2, the if statement is true and then next skips to the end of the loop, not executing anything in between, including the autoincrement of $i. Thus, $i will always stay at 2, and the loop will never exit. To get around this, you can use the optional continue statement:

```
while (TEST) {code block} continue {code block}
```

The code within the continue block is executed every time the loop is run, immediately after the termination of the loop code block no matter how the end of the code block was reached. So the safe way to deal with while loops that have next statements is to place the modification code in a continue block:

```
$i = 1;
while ($i < 50) {
  if (! $i%2) {next;}
  print "$i\n";
}
continue {
  $i++;
}
```

The last(), next(), and continue() functions can also be used independently of loops. A bare code block is the moral equivalent of a loop that executes once, so within that code block we can control the execution of that code block by jumping out of the block when we need to:

```
$gene = 'CFTR';
{
  if ($genetic{$gene} && $physical{$gene} && $rh{$gene}) {
    print "$gene is on all maps\n";
    last;
  }
  if ($genetic{$gene} && $physical{$gene}) {
    print "$gene is on genetic and physical maps\n";
```

```
        last;
    }
    if ($genetic{$gene} && $rh{$gene}) {
        print "$gene is on genetic and RH maps\n";
        last;
    }
    if ($physical{$gene} && $physical{$gene}) {
        print "$gene is on physical and RH maps\n";
        last;
    }
    print "$gene is not on multiple maps\n";
}
```

Finally, in some circumstances you may wish to go back and repeat the entire loop without modifying the loop control variable. The redo() function skips back up to the top of a for loop without evaluating the modification expression, thereby giving you a chance to try the loop over again. The redo function is illustrated in real use in Chapter 5.

Chapter Summary

- Comparison operators return Boolean values.
- A code block is a set of Perl statements enclosed in curly braces.
- The if, elsif, and else are used for conditional execution of a code block.
- For loops are determinate loops that execute a code block a set number of times.
- Foreach loops iterate over an array.
- While loops are indeterminate loops that execute a code block until a condition changes.
- Last, next, and continue add finer control to loop code structures.

Exercises

1. What type of loop would you use for each situation?

    a. printing an unknown number of sequences in a FASTA library

    b. incrementing each value of an array

    c. incrementing a counter

    d. listing all the values in an array

2. One of the many mantras of Perl programming is "There's more than one way to do it." Come up with as many ways as you can to create an indeterminate loop that executes at least once.

3. Do the following statements evaluate to true or false?

    a. 1

    b. 0 && 1

    c. 0||1

    d. 45

    e. 45 − 45

    f. 45/45

    g. 45==45

    h. 45 <=> 45

4. Explain the difference between determinate and indeterminate loops.

5. Differentiate between prematurely exiting a loop with the next and the last functions.

Programming Challenges

1. A control structure that many languages have that is not explicitly provided in Perl is the case (or switch) statement:

    ```
    switch (Variable) {
         case(Condition1): {code block 1}
         case(condition2): {code block 2}
    }
    ```

    Write a case statement emulator.

2. Write a determinate loop that prints out all the values in the %genetic hash.

3. Write an indeterminate loop that prints out all the values in the %genetic hash.

Part II

Intermediate Perl

Chapter 5

Subroutines

As your programs become more and more complex, you'll find yourself repeating the same chunk of code in multiple places within the same program. For example, you might end up computing the square root of several numbers in several different places when you're writing a statistical program that does an analysis of variance calculation on your data.

Fortunately, Perl has anticipated that and provided the sqrt() function, which can be used over and over. However, Perl is a relatively generic language, and not all instances where it would be useful to have a dedicated function have been anticipated. Therefore, Perl provides the subroutine as a generic mechanism to write reusable functions specific to your application.

5.1 Creating a Subroutine

A subroutine is a named code block that performs a specific task. The code block is set off by the keyword sub followed by the name and the code block:

```
sub NAME {code block}
```

The contents of the subroutine code block are not evaluated until the subroutine is invoked, so the subroutine can be placed anywhere in the script. However, it is common practice to place all the subroutines at the end of the file, after the end of the main script.

Subroutines are invoked by using either the & operator or by writing the name of the subroutine followed by the argument list. The latter is the preferred

Perl Programming for Biologists,   D. Curtis Jamison
ISBN 0-471-43059-5   Copyright © 2003 Wiley-Liss, Inc.

method. Simply write

```
NAME();
```

in your script, and the code block within subroutine NAME will be evaluated. So, for example, we might write a subroutine to print out a random sequence, 40 bp long. We would write:

```
sub RandomSeq {
  for ($i = 0; $i < 40; $i++) {
    $base = int(rand(4));
    if ($base == 0) {print "a"; next;}
    if ($base == 1) {print "c"; next;}
    if ($base == 2) {print "t"; next;}
    if ($base == 3) {print "g"; next;}
  }
  print "\n";
}
```

(The rand(EXPR) function returns a floating point number between 0 and the value of the EXPR, and the int() function turns it into and integer). Now, in the main program every time we used the statement

```
RandomSeq();
```

the program would print a 40-base long sequence. Note that as a matter of convention, the name of the subroutine is descriptive of what it does, and the first letter of every word is capitalized. This convention varies, with some people preferring all capital letters, and some people not caring. It really is a matter of personal preference, and this is the way I prefer.

5.2   Arguments

As useful as the ability to create simple subroutines like RandomSeq might be, the real power of Perl functions is the ability to pass values to them and have a value returned. We'd like our user-defined subroutines to have the same power. Thus, as you might expect, a subroutine can take and return values.

Values passed to a subroutine are called arguments. Arguments are passed to a subroutine by placing them in a list following the subroutine call. Perl takes the list and creates a temporary array called @_ which can be accessed from within the subroutine. For example, we can modify the RandomSeq subroutine to print a variable length sequence:

```
sub RandomSeq {
  $length = $_[0];
  for ($i = 0; $i < $length; $i++) {
    $base = int(rand(4));
    if ($base == 0) {print "a"; next;}
    if ($base == 1) {print "c"; next;}
    if ($base == 2) {print "t"; next;}
```

```
        if ($base == 3) {print "g"; next;}
    }
    print "\n";
}
```

and we then invoke it like so:

```
RandomSeq(30);
```

Now our subroutine is a little more flexible. The first thing we do is retrieve the value for how long the sequence should be. Because the arguments are passed in using the @_ array, the $_[0] slot contains the first value passed to the subroutine. The next step is to use that value to control a for loop to print out the specified number of bases.

A few more tweaks will make our subroutine complete (and illustrate a couple other points):

```
sub RandomSeq {
    $length = shift || 40;
    for ($i = 0; $i < $length; $i++) {
        unless ($i%70) {print "\n"};
        $base = int(rand(4));
        if ($base == 0) {print "a"; next;}
        if ($base == 1) {print "c"; next;}
        if ($base == 2) {print "t"; next;}
        if ($base == 3) {print "g"; next;}
    }
    print "\n";
}
```

First, notice how the script gets the length. We've used the shift operator and a short-circuit || operator to choose what value we use for length. Note that we didn't specify an array for the shift() operator. Because passing arguments to subroutines is such a common practice, the default array the shift operator uses @_ in a subroutine.

As for the short-circuit, remember that the || operator first evaluates the expression on the left, and quits if it is nonzero. So, if shift returns a value we will use that, otherwise the || operator uses 40. We now have defined a default value for our sequence length: if we invoke RandomSeq without a value the subroutine uses the default value of 40.

Finally, we added a line that checks to see whether our array counter is divisible by 70, meaning that we have printed out 70 characters. Because 70 characters is the default line length for a FASTA file, we put a new line in and go on to print the next character.

5.3 Return

Now we have a relatively useful subroutine for printing out random sequences, but what if we wanted a random sequence for use within the main body of our program? For that we would have to use the return() function. The return() function takes an argument and passes it back to the main program, where it can be assigned to a variable. If we wanted to use our subroutine in an assignment expression like

```
$mySeq = RandomSeq(80);
```

we could do it by making a few minor changes to our subroutine

```
sub RandomSeq {
  $length = shift || 40;
  $retval = "";
  for ($i = 0; $i < $length; $i++) {
    $base = int(rand(4));
    if ($base == 0) {$retval .= "a"; next;}
    if ($base == 1) {$retval .= "c"; next;}
    if ($base == 2) {$retval .= "t"; next;}
    if ($base == 3) {$retval .= "g"; next;}
    redo;
  }
  return $retval;
}
```

First, we've added a new variable called $retval, which we will use to hold a string containing our sequence as we generate it. Next, we replaced the print statements with the string append operator . = which adds the character string on the right to the end of the string on the left. We also did away with the lines that printed out the line returns. Finally, at the end of the subroutine we added the return statement, which causes Perl to pass back the value in $retval to the program.

Strictly speaking, using the return() function is not absolutely necessary. Without a return() statement, Perl uses the value of the last expression evaluated as the return value. So we could simply have written

```
$retval;
```

as the last line of the subroutine and allowed Perl to return that value for us. Some programmers prefer this abbreviated mechanism, because using the return function has a little more overhead in time and efficiency. However, while you'll see that usage in some scripts, using an explicit return function makes the code a little more readable and is worth the minor overhead costs to improve the readability of your program.

5.3.1 Wantarray

The return value of a subroutine is evaluated in the correct context as an array or scalar. This means that you typically don't have to worry about the return value too much, unless you want the subroutine to return specifically different things in the different contexts. The wantarray() function returns a Boolean value TRUE if the subroutine was called in an array context and FALSE if it was called in a scalar context:

```
if (wantarray) {
   return @arrayResult;
} else {
   return $scalarResult;
}
```

5.4   Scope

Variables in Perl default to being global. That is, after a variable is created it can be used anywhere in the script. To Perl, it doesn't really matter where a variable was created, or where it is being used. However, it often matters to the programmer.

For example, if we used our RandomSeq() subroutine, we could write code that accessed the internal variables:

```
$mySeq = RandomSeq(30);
print $retval;
```

which would print out the sequence we created and stored in $retval.

Things are even more dicey going in the opposite direction. If a variable is created before the subroutine is called, the variable is visible and usable inside the subroutine. Any changes to the variable inside the subroutine are reflected outside the subroutine. So

```
$length = 500;
print "before subroutine, length is $length\n";
$mySeq = RandomSeq;
print "after subroutine, length is $length\n";
```

produces the output

```
before subroutine, length is 500
after subroutine, length is 40
```

because we used the length variable inside the RandomSeq subroutine, and it changed the value of $length. If we were using $length for something important in the outer code block, we'd have a small problem.

5.4.1   My

Variables that are visible throughout the program are called global variables. Usually global variables are undesirable, because they can lead to subtle errors and bugs in the program. Perl allows you to circumvent global variable definitions by the use of the my() command. Putting the word my in front of a variable restricts the use of the variable to the current code block (and embedded) code blocks, while making it invisible to the rest of the program, including any subroutines called from the current code block. So

```
{
  my $length = 500;
  print "before subroutine, length is $length\n";
  $mySeq = RandomSeq;
  print "after subroutine, length is $length\n";
}
```

produces

```
before subroutine, length is 500
after subroutine, length is 500
```

Note that we put in the curly braces to ensure that the my statement falls within a code block.

While this works, it is actually a better idea to put the my command into the subroutine:

```
sub RandomSeq {
  my $length = shift || 40;
  my $retval = "";
  for (my $i = 0; $i < $length; $i++) {
    my $base = int(rand(4));
    if ($base == 0) {$retval .= "a"; next;}
    if ($base == 1) {$retval .= "c"; next;}
    if ($base == 2) {$retval .= "t"; next;}
    if ($base == 3) {$retval .= "g"; next;}
    redo;
  }
  return $retval;
}
```

That way, it doesn't matter if the outside world uses the same variable names as found inside the subroutine, because the my command limits the scope of any subroutine variables to inside the subroutine itself.

It typically is a good idea to use code blocks and the my command liberally in all your subroutines. This will not only protect you from making errors in your own code, but it will protect your variables from unruly subroutines you might access in other people's modules. The structure I like to use in my large-scale Perl programs is

```
#!/path/to/Perl

# opening comments go here

# any global variables go here

{
    # main code block goes here
}

# any subroutines go here
```

So, the file I've been using for the subroutine example looks like

```
#!/usr/bin/perl

## program to illustrate subroutines
## cjamison@gmu.edu
## 20July2001

use strict;

{
  my $length = 500;
  print "before subroutine, length is $length\n";
  my $mySeq =  RandomSeq;
  print "after subroutine, length is $length\n";
}

sub RandomSeq {
  my $length = shift || 40;
  my $retval = "";
  for (my $i = 0; $i < $length; $i++) {
    my $base = int(rand(4));
    if ($base == 0) {$retval .= "a"; next;}
    if ($base == 1) {$retval .= "c"; next;}
    if ($base == 2) {$retval .= "t"; next;}
    if ($base == 3) {$retval .= "g"; next;}
  }
  return $retval;
}
```

The opening comments provide a quick commentary on what the code is supposed to do, who wrote it, and when. Any later code modifications would warrant a few lines about the changes. The use strict is a directive that loads the strict Perl module (see Chapter 8) that warns you when you use global variables or otherwise deviate from good Perl coding practices. Finally, any subroutines are placed after the main code block.

Although this version of our program has no global variables, it does illustrate a situation where one could prove useful. Global variables should be used for values that keep cropping up and are needed by every subroutine. Generally, these values are constants like pi or the four nucleotides. For example, we could rewrite our random sequence program to use a global array to hold the values of the nucleotides:

```
#!/usr/bin/perl

## program to illustrate subroutines
## cjamison@gmu.edu
## 20July2001

@nucleotides = ('a','c','g','t');
```

```
MAIN: {
  my $length = 500;
  print "before subroutine, length is $length\n";
  my $mySeq = RandomSeq;
  print "after subroutine, length is $length\n";
}

sub RandomSeq {
  my $length = shift || 40;
  my $retval = "";
  for (my $i = 0; $i < $length; $i++) {
    my $base = $nucleotides[int(rand(4))];
    if (!$base) {redo;}
    $retval .= $base;
  }
  return $retval;
}
```

The advantage of using a global variable in this case is that we can alter the nucleotide array and have the change available to the entire program. So if we were to change the 't' to a 'u', we will have changed the program from creating a DNA sequence to an RNA sequence. While admittedly in this simple example the maintenance cost-savings of this approach is minimal because we only use the nucleotide array in one place, imagine the savings if we had several dozen subroutines, all of which needed to deal with the nucleotide array. Instead of having to find a myriad of places where we used a 't', we now change one line and it propagates through the code. This approach is called generic programming, and we'll see more of it in Chapter 10 when we talk about object-oriented programming.

5.5   Passing Arguments with References

One difficulty with using subroutines is passing arrays. Subroutine arguments are passed as lists, and when Perl sees array variable names in a list context it flattens them out into a list. For example, if we were to write:

```
@array1 = ('a', 'b', 'c');
@array2 = ('d', 'e', 'f');
arrayroutine(@array1, @array2);
```

the two arrays would get flattened into a single list

```
('a', 'b', 'c', 'd', 'e', 'f')
```

and our array routine would have no idea how to separate them into the two original lists. Although we could add scalars at the beginning of each array telling the array routine how to separate the arrays, the subroutine becomes more complex at the beginning as it tries to read the variables:

```
@array1 = ('a', 'b', 'c');
@array2 = ('d', 'e', 'f');
arrayroutine($#array1, @array1, $#array2, @array2);

sub arrayroutine {
  $lastindex = shift;
  for ($i = 0; $i <= $lastindex; $i++) {
      my $array1[$i] = shift;
  }
  $lastindex = shift;
  for ($i = 0; $i <= $lastindex; $i++) {
      my $array2[$i] = shift;
  }
  ...
```

Although this works, we're limited to knowing exactly how many arrays are being passed, and generalizing the array reading method will be even more complex. Fortunately, there is a simpler way. We can create a reference to the array to pass to the routine. We do this by prepending the \ symbol to the array name and passing the reference to the subroutine. References are actually a special scalar data type, and so inside the subroutine we need to convert them back into local arrays. We would write:

```
@array1 = ('a', 'b', 'c');
@array2 = ('d', 'e', 'f');
arrayroutine(@array1, @array2);

sub arrayroutine {
  my ($ref1, $ref2) = @_;
  @a1 = @{$ref1};
  @a2 = @{$ref2};
  # now use @a1 and @a2 normally...
```

We'll see more of references in Chapter 9.

5.6 Sort Subroutines

The sort function that we used in Chapter 3 is a very interesting function. There we used the function put a list in order:

```
@alpha_list = sort(@genes);
```

which took the list in @ genes and returned a list sorted in alphabetical order. However, it was also noted that there was another form of the command, which took a user-defined subroutine to replace the standard alphabetical sorting routine.

The sort function works by taking two values in the list, comparing them, and then swapping them according to the signed comparison result. Specifically, the first value is placed in the $a variable, and the second is placed in the $b variable, and then the two variables are passed to the specified subroutine. If the value returned by the sorting subroutine is positive, the sort routine will swap the value of $a and $b, then return them to the array.

The default sorting behavior is to sort lexically, that is, using a straight string comparison like we would get using the cmp operator to compare two strings. In fact, the cmp operator is exactly what sort uses. The default behavior for sorting is exactly as if we had written

```
$a cmp $b
```

as a conditional expression. The cmp operator returns a positive value only if $a is greater than $b, and so the two values will be switched.

We can change the behavior of sort by providing a conditional to compare $a and $b in a manner that duplicates the way we want sort to behave. We place the conditional in a code block between the sort keyword and the argument list:

```
sort {conditional} (list)
```

So we can duplicate the default behavior of sort by writing

```
sort {$a cmp $b} (list)
```

or, to illustrate with our earlier example, we could write

```
@alpha_list = sort {$a cmp $b} (@genes);
```

and the list in @alpha_list will be the same as before (sorted in alphabetical order).

Let's suppose we wanted to sort in reverse alphabetical order. That is, we want to swap the two values if the second value is greater. To do so, we simply have to reverse our conditional and return a positive number when $b is greater than $a:

```
@rev_alpha_list = sort {$b cmp $a} (@genes);
```

Swapping the $a and $b variables simply reverses the meaning of the comparison, and thus results in a list in reverse alphabetical order.

We are not restricted to using the signed string comparison operator in our comparisons. Remember the idea of sorting a list of oligos by their length from Chapter 3. We can't do so using the default lexical search

```
@oligos = ('ATGCGTTG', 'GTAGG', 'TAGATGGATTC',
'ATTGA', 'CAGGATG');

@sorted = sort @oligos;
print join("\n", @sorted), "\n";
```

which simply prints the oligos sorted lexically by base:

```
ATGCGTTG
ATTGA
CAGGATG
GTAGG
TAGATGGATTC
```

However, we can insert a comparison that is based upon the length of the oligo, using the length function to calculate the length of the string:

```
@oligos = ('ATGCGTTG', 'GTAGG', 'TAGATGGATTC',
           'ATTGA', 'CAGGATG');

@sorted = sort {length($a) <=> length($b)} @oligos;
print join("\n", @sorted), "\n";
```

Note that because the length is a number, we use the numeric signed equality operator. Now the sort routine uses the length to produce the sorted list:

```
GTAGG
ATTGA
CAGGATG
ATGCGTTG
TAGATGGATTC
```

The search code can be arbitrarily complex. The only limitation is that it has to return a positive value when the two values need to be swapped. But if the code gets too complex, the readability of the code can suffer. Thus there is a third form of sort that accepts the name of a subroutine in place of the code block. To use this form, we simply create a subroutine that returns the results of the comparison:

```
@oligos = ('ATGCGTTG', 'GTAGG', 'TAGATGGATTC',
           'ATTGA', 'CAGGATG');

@sorted = sort byLength @oligos;
print join("\n", @sorted), "\n";

sub byLength {
  return (length($a) <=> length($b))
}
```

returns the same length-sorted list as before, but now it is immediately clear that we are sorting the list by length. The sorting subroutine is not passed any variables: $a and $b are created globally for it. However, this means that any accidental changes to $a or $b will be reflected in the values in list being sorted. Because changing the values as you sort the list is generally a bad idea, if your sort subroutine is very complex and performs calculations that could change the values, you should copy the values from $a and $b into variables that are locally scoped with the my command.

Chapter Summary

- A subroutine is a named block of code that can be used in multiple places.
- Subroutine arguments are passed via the @_ array.
- Subroutine results are passed back via the return() function.

- The wantarray() function checks whether the subroutine was used in an array context.
- The my command restricts the scope of variables.

For More Information

```
perldoc perlfunc
perldoc perlsub
```

Exercises

1. What is the difference between a Perl function and a Perl subroutine?
2. Passing an array to a subroutine expands the array into a list, which then gets assigned to the @_ variable. Give at least two ways of passing both an array and several scalars to a subroutine.
3. What is variable scope, and why is it important for subroutines?

Programming Challenges

1. Write a subroutine that multiplies an array of integers by a scalar value.
2. Write a subroutine that takes a hash and inverts the key-value pairs. (*Hint*: Hashes get flattened into a list of alternating key value pairs.)
3. Using one of the methods you defined in exercise 2, write a subroutine that multiplies every value of an array by a scalar.
4. Write a sorting subroutine that sorts oligos based upon their GC content.

Chapter 6

String Manipulation

The most useful aspect of Perl is the string manipulation capabilities built into the language. Perl provides both simple array-based character manipulation commands and mind-bogglingly powerful regular expression pattern matching and string manipulation commands. Together, these commands allow the programmer to search and transform strings with incredible ease, and is one of the primary reasons to choose Perl as a programming language.

6.1 Array-Based Character Manipulation

As their name implies, the array-based character manipulation commands treat a string as if it were an array of single characters. This is the model used by many other languages such as C and Fortran. An array-based view of a DNA sequence would look like Figure 6.1. Each slot of the array contains a single letter of the sequence, and the sequence can be manipulated using the indices associated with each letter.

Of course, strings are scalars, and the indices associated with each letter are an artificial external construct based the value of the string rather than an inherent characteristic of the data structure. Therefore, we need to use specialized commands to utilize the imaginary indices.

To get the index associated with a substring, we use the eponymous index() command:

```
index(STRING, SUBSTRING, POSITION)
```

Perl Programming for Biologists, D. Curtis Jamison
ISBN 0-471-43059-5   Copyright © 2003 Wiley-Liss, Inc.

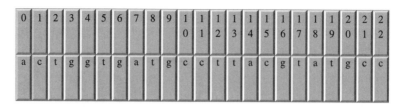

0	1	2	3	4	5	6	7	8	9	1 0	1 1	1 2	1 3	1 4	1 5	1 6	1 7	1 8	1 9	2 0	2 1	2 2
a	c	t	g	g	t	g	a	t	g	c	c	t	t	a	c	g	t	a	t	g	c	c

Figure 6.1 An array of characters

which takes the STRING and searches for the SUBSTRING starting from the specified POSITION. A good example of how to use the index command is the process of searching a long sequence for a start codon:

```
$seqStart = index($sequence, 'ATG');
```

In this example, we are looking through the string contained in $sequence for a string of letters corresponding to 'ATG'. The default value for the starting position is the beginning of the string, so we can safely leave it out. The number that ends up in $seqStart is the index of the character at the start of the match.

We can use the index and the POSITION variable to look through a genomic sequence for all start codons:

```
$position = 0;
while (($position = index($sequence, 'ATG', $position)) >= 0) {
  push(@seqStart, $position);
  $position++;
}
```

The expression controlling the while loop is true when there is an ATG in the sequence downstream of $position: index() returns −1 otherwise. The control expression also modifies $position to be the next index of ATG, which we push onto an array of start positions. Finally, we push our search start position ahead by one so we don't keeping finding the same ATG over and over again. Note that we start $position at 0: remember that strings are like arrays in that their numbering system begins at 0.

The index() command searches left to right. To search right to left, the completely analogous rindex is used to look for start codons in the reverse strand:

```
$position = length($sequence);
while (($position = rindex($sequence, 'CAT', $position)) >= 0) {
  push(@seqStart, $position);
  $position--;
}
```

In this code, there are three changes. First, we are using rindex() to search from right to left so we autodecrement the position. We also reverse complemented our search string, changing it from 'ATG' to 'CAT'. And finally, we used the length() command to give us the starting position (the far right end).

Often we want to extract a portion of a string. We can create a new string by excising a chunk from an existing string using the substr() command:

```
substr(STRING, START, LENGTH)
```

The substr() command returns a new string excised from STRING, beginning at START and running for LENGTH characters. If START is negative, substr begins counting from the end of STRING. So, if we wanted to store the first 60 nucleotides following the start codons in our genomic sequence, we could write

```
$position = 0;
while (($position = index($sequence, 'ATG', $position)) >= 0) {
  push(@seqs, substr($sequence, $position, 60));
  $position++;
}
```

If the sum of the START and LENGTH arguments is greater then the length of the original, the new string will run from START to the end of the original sequence. Similarly, if the LENGTH argument is omitted, the default length is from the position specified by the START argument to the end of the original sequence.

The substr() command is relatively versatile. It can also be used to splice characters into a string by placing it on the left side of the assignment:

```
$string = "my short string";
substr($string, 3, 0) = "not so ";
print $string, "\n";
```

results in

```
my not so short string
```

The string on the right has been inserted into $string, which grows in response. The substr() command has started at position 3 and replaced the substring of length 0 with the string on the right. In addition to inserting, we can actually replace portions:

```
substr($string, 3, 5) = "long and convoluted example";
```

replaces the word "short" in the original string and results in

```
my long and convoluted example string
```

The substr() command can be used to append or prepend strings by using a start index of 0 or length(), respectively, and then using a 0 for the length argument. A simpler and faster way to do so is to use the concatenation operator, which is the . symbol. This operator takes the strings on either side and creates a single string by appending the string on the right to the string on the left:

```
$newstring = "new" . "string";
```

We have already seen this operator in action with the concatenation assignment operator:

```
$retval .= $base;
```

which is the short-hand equivalent of

```
$retval = $retval . $base;
```

There are two major caveats to remember when working with array-based character operators. First, there is a special Perl variable defined that can alter the numbering system of the character indices. Certain misguided programmers, in an attempt to make Perl act more like inferior programming languages, will change the value of the starting index so that the Perl commands work more like the ones they are used to. In general, this qualifies as a very bad idea, and if you come across code that has done this, it is best to throw it away and start all over again because you can't be sure of what other atrocities the programmer has committed.

The second caveat is much more likely to rear up and bite unsuspecting novice programmers. Perl (and computers in general) treat all characters as equal, whether or not the character is seen when it is sent to the printer. Thus, a newline character "\n" counts as a character when querying the length of a string. So does a space or a tab character.

Typically, one runs into newlines when reading text from a file. Because this is a very common problem, Perl has the chomp() command:

```
chomp ($VAR)
chomp (LIST)
chomp
```

The chomp command removes the character at the end of the string if it matches the character stored in the special variable $/ (known as the record input separator, it is set to "\n" by default). If chomp is given a LIST, it removes the trailing $/ character string from each string in the list. The default variable that chomp works on is the $_ variable, which we will see in great detail next. A multipurpose variable, $_ is the default target for all text operations, including character-based methods, regular expression searches, and file input.

6.2   Regular Expressions

As powerful as the array-based character manipulation commands are, they pale in comparison to the regular expression operators. These operators perform pattern matching using regular expressions, and can be used to search, substitute, and transform strings of any length. Regular expressions can be daunting, because they often look like they were composed by a random short-circuit from the keyboard, but once you get the hang of them they become almost second nature, and they serve as one of the key foundations of Perl programming.

There are only four regular expression operators. They are

```
[m]/PATTERN/[g][i][o]
s/PATTERN/PATTERN]/[g][i][e][o]
tr/PATTERNLIST/PATTERNLIST/[c][d][s]
y/PATTERNLIST/PATTERNLIST/[c][d][s]
```

These operators look a little odd, because they were inherited from other programming languages, and have retained their old-fashioned appearance, but they work exactly like any of the comparison operators and functions: they take arguments, perform a task, and return a value.

The m operator is the match operator. It looks for the PATTERN in a string. The s operator is the substitute operator, and it finds the first PATTERN and replaces it with the second PATTERN. Finally, the tr and y operators are synonymous, taking a PATTERN from the first PATTERNLIST and replacing it with the corresponding PATTERN from the second PATTERNLIST.

Both the return value and the behavior of each operator can be modified by one or more optional switches:

```
[c]omplement
[d]elete
[e]valuate
[g]lobal
[i]nsensitive to case
[o]nly evaluate once
[s]queeze multiple characters
```

In practice, the g and i switches are typically the most useful, and the others are very rarely seen. And, of course, the return value is modified by whether you are using the regular expression operator in a scalar or an array context.

By default, the regular expression operators use the $_ variable to get the string value to work with. Because $_ is the default variable for reading from files and any other operation that produces a string value, the default is typically quite useful. For example:

```
if (m/ATG/) {print "Start codon found\n";}
```

looks at the string in $_ and returns true or false. However, the string we want to search in often isn't in the $_ variable. Rather than assigning the string into the $_ variable, we can make the match operators use a different variable as the target string by using the =~ operator:

```
$mySeq = RandomSeq(250);
if ($mySeq =~ m/ATG/) {print "Start codon found\n";}
```

In practice, your code will almost always be clearer to understand if you assign the target string into a variable and use the =~ operator.

6.2.1 Match

The match operator will return a 1 if it is used in a scalar context (such as a loop conditional). Thus, in the example above, when we looked through the string in

$mySeq, the match operator returned either a true or a false value depending on if it found any start codons.

On the other hand, we might want to know how many start codons are in the sequence. To do this, we can take advantage of the fact that when the match operator is used in an array context with the [g]lobal option, it will return an array of the pattern matches:

```
$mySeq = RandomSeq(250);
@starts = $mySeq =~ m/ATG/g;
print "sequence has" . $#starts . "start codons\n";
```

While the second line looks rather strange, it really is not very difficult to understand. The trick is that the =~ operator and the match operator have a higher precedence than the assignment operator. Thus, the expression on the left side of the assignment operator is evaluated first, with the [g]lobal option causing the match operator to find all the occurrences of "ATG" in $mySeq, and then creating a list out of them because of the array context. Then we simply use the $# notation to count how many items are in the @starts array.

The regular expression operators will only produce a list if the [g]lobal switch is used in an array context. If the operator is used in a scalar context, the operators will only return 1 or the undef value. Similarly, even if the operator is used in an array context, it will only return 1 or the undef value if the [g]lobal option has been omitted. In the latter case, we get an array of length one that contains either a 1 or the undef value as the first value.

The match operator is used so commonly that Perl has given us a shortcut. It turns out the leading m is optional, and any pattern between two forward slashes tells Perl to perform the match. Thus we could have written our start codon matching code as

```
@starts = $mySeq =~ /ATG/g;
```

and gotten the same result. Most Perl programmers will omit the m.

However, there is a downside to the shortcut. If there are forward slashes in the pattern you are trying to match (like a Unix directory path, for example), they will interfere with the regular expression. To get around this, you can use any pair of nonalphanumeric characters as the pattern delimiters along with the m:

```
m#/usr/local/bin#
```

will match any line containing the Unix path to a particular directory.

If the pattern contains a pattern that looks like it might contain a variable, Perl attempts to interpolate the variable to create the pattern. So we can make our matching pattern easier to change (at the cost of some clarity and performance) by setting a variable to contain the search string:

```
$mySeq = RandomSeq(250);
$myStart = "ATG";
push (@starts, $mySeq =~ /$myStart/g);
print "sequence has" . $#starts . "start codons\n";
```

In addition to the [g]lobal switch, the match operator also accepts the [i]nsensitive, which makes all matches in a case-insensitive manner, and the [o]nce switch, which causes any variable interpolation within the pattern to occur only once, which can save much time in loops.

6.2.2   Substitute

The substitute operator is useful for performing large-scale search and replacement. For example, we might want to change our DNA sequence to an RNA sequence:

```
$mySeq = RandomSeq(250);
$mySeq =~ s/T/U/g;
```

This code tells Perl to take the string and replace every T with a U. Like the match operator, we can specify that the substitution take place [g]lobally. We can also use the i and the o switch with the same meanings as before.

A new switch for the substitute operator is the [e]valuate switch. This tells Perl that the replacement pattern is an expression, and the expression should be evaluated before the replacement. To illustrate, we can make our DNA to RNA transcription code a little more complex:

```
$newCodon = 'U';
$mySeq = RandomSeq(250);
$mySeq =~ s/T/$newCodon/eg;
```

Note that when using options, it doesn't matter in what order they appear.

6.2.3   Translate

Perl has two translation operators: tr and y. The two are exactly equivalent, and the reasons for having both lie back in the prehistory of Perl and the language *sed*, from which many of the regular expression syntax derives. For new Perl programmers the tr operator is easier and more sensible to remember.

The tr operator takes the characters in the first pattern and replaces them with the characters in the second pattern. The first character in the matching pattern list is replaced with the first character in the replacement pattern list, the second with the second, and so forth. This is very different from the substitute operator, which assumes that the entire matching pattern is to be replaced with the entire replacement pattern.

A perfect example of using the translate function is to reverse complement a sequence:

```
$mySeq = RandomSeq(250);
$mySeq =~ tr/ACTG/TGAC/;
$revcomp = reverse($mySeq);
```

Using the reverse function on a string returns a reversed string, analogous to using reverse on an array that contained a single letter in each slot.

Also, note that we did not use the [g]lobal option. The tr operator always acts globally. There are three switches that can be used with the tr operator. The [c]omplement switch inverses the search list, interpreting the list as containing every possible character *except* those listed in the search list. Thus

```
tr/ACTG/ /c;
```

replaces every character that is not an A, C, G, or T with a space, which could be a very useful device for cleaning uncertainty characters out of a sequence. Note that the replacement list is shorter than the search list: in cases like this Perl reuses the last character in the replacement list. Be careful not to confuse the [c]omplement option with the biological meaning of nucleic acid complement.

Another switch is the [s]queeze option, which will compress a run of replacement characters into a single character. Thus, if you have a sequence like

```
ACTGGTAxxxxxxxATAGGxxTGAT
```

the command

```
tr/ACTG/ /cs;
```

would result in the string

```
ACTGGTA ATAGG TGAT
```

The tr operator returns a scalar value stating how many replacements were made. If we had assigned the last tr command to a scalar, the variable would have contained 9 as the number of x's we replaced. We can make use of this to count symbols if we make the replacement list the same as the search list:

```
$hydrophobic = tr/TFY/TFY/;
```

would count the number of hydrophobic residues in a protein sequence without actually altering the sequence. Because this is a common task, as we would expect, Perl provides a shortcut to reduce our typing. Leaving out the replacement list causes the search list to be replicated as the replacement list, so we could have written our residue counter as

```
$hydrophobic = tr/TFY//;
```

with no change in meaning. Which brings us to our last switch, the [d]elete switch, which causes any matches to be removed completely:

```
tr/ACTG//cd;
```

causes all the uncertainty codes in our first example to be removed completely.

6.3 Patterns

Thus far, we've begged off a bit on the question of exactly what a pattern is. A pattern is composed of a set of atoms, quantifiers, and assertions. Atoms are the individual characters that make up the pattern, quantifiers are phrases that control how many atoms are seen, and assertions control where the atoms are found. Together, the three aspects of patterns make for an incredibly rich and powerful language.

6.3.1   Atoms

We've seen some examples of patterns that are simple character strings. The character string represents a series of atoms, which are the basic single character matching substrate. For example, when searching for the start codon, we created a pattern of three atoms: A, T, and G. The regular expression operator then looked for those three atoms in the specified order.

Any character that Perl recognizes can be used as an atom. That includes letters, numbers, and spaces. Each character matches itself once, unless it is quantified. Characters protected with a backslash match that character, with the following exceptions:

- \c followed by a character matches the corresponding control character. For example, \cD matches the Control-D character;

- \x followed by a two-digit hexadecimal number matches the character having that hexadecimal value;

- \0 used as a two- or three-digit octal value matches the character with that octal value;

- \n matches a newline;

- \r matches a return;

- \f matches a form feed;

- \t matches a tab;

- \d, \D, \w, \W, \s, \S match special character classes defined below.

6.3.2   Special Atoms

Certain characters and combinations of characters create special complex atoms. Complex atoms can be combined with quantifiers and assertions just like regular atoms. The only trick is that if you want to match on one of these special characters rather than using it as a complex atom, you have to backslash-escape the character.

A . matches any character except the \n character. So the pattern

    A.G

matches ATG, ACG, AAG, and AGG, as well as any other triplet of letters that starts with A and ends with G. You can restrict the atom by giving a list of characters in square brackets:

```
A[ATCG]G
```

will match only valid nucleotide triplets and ignores any triplets that have nonvalid DNA characters.

A hyphen between two characters in square brackets specifies a range of characters to look for. So

```
[0-9]
```

would match any digit in that range. Similarly,

```
[a-z]
```

matches any lowercase letter, and

```
[a-zA-Z]
```

matches any letter no matter what case it is. A ˆ at the front of the list negates the class:

```
[ˆa-z]
```

matches any character that is not a lowercase letter.

Some ranges are so useful that Perl defines some backslash-escaped characters that match a specific class

- \d matches any digit, the same as [0–9]
- \D matches any nondigit, the same as [ˆ0–9]
- \w matches any alphanumeric character, the same as [0-9a-zA-Z]
- \W matches any nonalphanumeric character, the same as [ˆ0-9a-zA-Z]
- \s matches any white-space character, the same as [\t\n\r\f]
- \S matches any non-white-space character, the same as [\ˆ \t\n\r\f]

Note that \w is not equivalent to \S, and \W is not equivalent to \s. This is because there are symbol and control characters that won't match the \w or \s atom, but will match the \W and \S atom.

6.3.3 Quantifiers

Atoms can be quantified, meaning that a specific number of the atoms must be present. Quantifiers are placed directly behind the atom they are quantifying. The general syntax is

```
{x,y}
```

where x and y are numbers. The quantifier indicates the atom must be matched at least x times but not more than y times. Thus

    A{100,200}

would match runs of at least 100 and no more than 200 A's (the definition of valid polyadenylations) in a file of mRNA sequences.

Leaving the second argument undefined

    {x,}

means the math must occur at least x times, but there is no upper limit. Providing only the first argument

    {x}

means the match must occur exactly x times. Note the difference between the two is the presence of the comma: with a comma the second argument is undefined, whereas without it the second argument is deleted.

Not surprisingly, Perl has several special case quantifier symbols defined for commonly used quantifiers:

- * matches 0 or more times, same as {0,}

- + matches 1 or more times, same as {1,}

- ? matches 0 or 1 times, same as {0,1}

6.3.4 Assertions

Finally, the regular expression language is rounded out by four assertions that control where the matches are located. The ˆ symbol matches the beginning of the string, the $ symbol matches the end of the string, a \b matches at a word boundary, and a \B matches at a nonword boundary. Note that the ˆ and the $ have other meanings as well, and it is important to check the context of the symbol:

    $seq =~ /^[AUCG]*A{100, 200}$/

is a way to validate that $seq contains a mRNA sequence, whereas

    $seq =~ /[^AUCG]*A{100, 200}$/

makes sure there are no A, U, C, or G characters in the match, which more than likely is not what the programmer intended.

6.3.5 Alternatives

Often we run across situations where multiple patterns are valid. For example, if we wanted to look for start codons in bacteria, we should take into account the fact that some species have alternative start codons. We could look twice (or more) using the Boolean OR operator:

```
if (($seq =~ /AUG/) || ($seq =~ /AGG/)) {...}
```

but that is somewhat unwieldy. Perl allows us to collapse the alternatives into a single regular expression by using the | symbol (half an OR):

```
if ($seq =~ /(AUG)|(AGG)/) {...}
```

Any number of alternatives can be separated by the | symbol. Alternatives are evaluated left to right and the evaluation stops on the first positive match, much like the || command.

The parentheses serve to consolidate individual atoms into a single larger atom. This is useful if we want to more create complex matching schemes. For example, we might want to look for CAG expansion repeats in our DNA sequence:

```
/((CAG)+)/
```

The parentheses also have another beneficial side effect. They can be used to extract the last string that matched the expression inside the parentheses. Each pair of parentheses associated with either a + or a * is assigned a number, going from left to right, and a variable consisting of the $ and the assigned number of the parentheses is created to contain the match. Thus, if we used our expression for real, $1 would contain the first CAG expansion matched in the sequence:

```
my $rna = 'UAAGACGUCAGCAGCAGCAGCAGAAAAGCAGCAGAAA';
if ($rna =~ /((CAG)+)/) {
  print "The first expansion is $1 \n";
}
```

which will produce:

```
The first expansion is CAGCAGCAGCAGCAG
```

The numbered variables aren't the only ones created by the regular expression operator. The $ variable contains the entire matched string, whereas $` and $' return everything before and after the match respectively. These variables are scoped to the block that contains the regular expression, so that they cannot be accessed or are changed back to their original status after the block is finished. These variables are undefined if a match is not found.

Chapter Summary

- Array-based character manipulation treats a character string like an array of characters.

- Exact string matches can be found using the index() and rindex() commands.

- Substrings can be extracted using the substr() command.
- Regular expressions use pattern matching to manipulate strings.
- The m operator finds pattern matches.
- The s operator substitutes a string for a pattern.
- The tr and y operators translate one pattern list into another pattern list.
- The $_ variable is the default target for regular expression operators.
- The =~ operator causes the regular expression operator to act upon the string in the variable on the left.

For More Information

```
perldoc perlfunc
perldoc perlre
```

Exercises

1. Write a subroutine that performs the same function as the chop() command.
2. Compare and contrast Prosite motifs to Perl regular expressions.
3. Write a regular expression that will find GAG repeat expansions.
4. Write a regular expression that represents prokaryotic translation start sites.
5. Give examples of when to use the array-based character manipulation commands versus the regular expression commands.
6. Write a subroutine that duplicates the function of the regular expression s/// operator using array-based character manipulation commands. Take into account wild-cards and identifiers.

Programming Challenges

1. A common use of Perl is to read a tab- or space-delimited file into an array, and then manipulate the results. For example, many microarray programs leave the data in Excel spreadsheets that can be exported to tab-delimited text files:

```
Number      Name   ch1_Ratio    ch1_Percent ch2_Ratio
      ch2_Percent
1     Mouse_actin_beta   1     43.366182    1.305944
      56.633818
2     cytochrome_P450_2b9    1     60.364437    0.656605
      39.635563
```

```
3       thrombomodulin    1    51.152543   0.954937
        48.847457
4       cytokine_inducible_protein      1      50.155169
        0.993812    49.844831
5       Glvr-1_mRNA_complete_cds        1      46.36159
        1.156958    53.63841
6       PDE1A2       1    47.743435   1.094529    52.256565
7       Fas-associated_factor_1 1      46.01072    1.173407
        53.98928
```

Write a program that parses the information out of files with this format and print out the gene names and fold-differences in descending order.

2. Write a program that splices out introns from a sequence.

3. Write a program that translates an RNA sequence to a protein sequence, keeping track of codon usage.

Chapter 7

Input and Output

Programs with encoded values are necessarily of limited value due their inflexible nature. For example, when we defined the arrays of genes and map positions in Chapter 3, we put the values of the genes and map positions directly into the program, a process known as hard-coding. Hard-coding data values limits the flexibility and utility of the program. Although such programs are often sufficient, a much better approach would be the ability to input the information the program needs at the time we run the program, so the same code can be used over and over again in different situations with different data (*e.g.*, a chromosome 6 gene list rather than a chromosome 7 gene list).

Perl provides two mechanisms for getting information into programs. In the simplest case, we can pass parameters and arguments to the program. In a more complex case, we can use filehandles to read and write information to and from files. Program parameters work well for simple, short arguments than can easily be typed on the command line, whereas filehandles work better when the data sets are large. Typically, both methods are used, using a program parameter to specify a file name for a filehandle.

7.1 Program Parameters

Parameters can be passed to a Perl script in a manner similar to that used to pass arguments to a subroutine. On the Unix command line, a list of space-separated values follows the Perl script name:

```
haydn 2% myscript.pl arg1 arg2 arg3
```

which gives three arguments into the program.

Perl Programming for Biologists, D. Curtis Jamison
ISBN 0-471-43059-5 Copyright © 2003 Wiley-Liss, Inc.

Inside the Perl script, we need to deal with converting the parameters into variables we can use. Fortunately, Perl does most of the work for us by creating a special array variable called @ARGV (the name derives from C, and stands for ARGument Values). The @ARGV array contains the command line parameters converted from a list to an array.

The @ARGV array can be treated like a normal array. Thus $ARGV[0] is the first parameter, and $#ARGV is the index of the last parameter passed into the program. It is useful to check the latter and make sure that the proper number of variables have been passed into the program:

```
unless ($#ARGV == 2) {
  die "usage: $1 arg1 arg2 arg3\n";
}
```

Thus, if we tried to run myscript with only two arguments, the program would issue a gentle reminder:

```
haydn 3% myscript.pl arg1 arg2
usage: myscript.pl arg1 arg2 arg3
haydn  4%
```

Because @ARGV is a normal array, we can assign it directly to a variable list:

```
($var1, $var2, $var3) = @ARGV;
```

Sometimes we don't know exactly how many parameters will be passed from the command line. In that case, we can use the shift() command like we did in the subroutines. In fact, in the main block of the program, @ARGV, is the default target of the shift() command, so we don't have to specify it as an argument:

```
while ($value = shift) {
  ## process value
}
```

Command line argument processing can be greatly facilitated by using the Getopt Perl module, now part of the standard Perl distribution (see Chapter 8).

7.2   File I/O

7.2.1   Filehandles

Getting large amounts data in and out of a program can sometimes be a challenge. Most programs need some sort of input to get the data to start with, and every program needs to output results. The Perl input and output (I/O) commands make getting information in and out relatively easy.

We have seen the basic Perl output operator, the print command, several times thus far. The operation seems pretty simple: print takes a string and writes it out on the screen. Although this is essentially correct, there is one more level of complexity that makes the print statement incredibly powerful.

All Perl I/O takes place using an data structure called a filehandle. The name is pretty much descriptive of the function, which is to provide a handle that we use to gain access to a file. In practice, a filehandle is simply a name that has been associated with a particular file using the open() command:

```
open(filehandle, filename)
```

The filehandle is just an unquoted string like INPUT or FILE. Although it is not required, most Perl programmers put filehandles in all capital letters to make them readily distinguishable from the rest of the program code. The filename is a string containing the name of the file, including whatever directory path information is needed for Perl to find the input file. At the front of the name is a symbol indicating how we wish to open the file: a < symbol opens the file for reading, the > file opens the file for writing (wiping out the previous contents, if any), and >> open the file for appending. Adding a + symbol in front of the > or < symbol opens the file for both reading and writing.

7.2.2 Working with Files

The difference between opening a file for writing and opening a file for appending must be emphasized. If a file opened for writing already exists, the contents of that file are replaced with the output of the program. Appending, on the other hand, simply adds the program output to the end of the file. If the file doesn't exist, open will create the file (in either mode). So, if we had a file that looked like

```
haydn 7% more text.txt
the quick red fox

haydn 8%
```

the code

```
open (APPEND, ">>text.txt");
print APPEND "jumped over\n";
```

would result in the file

```
haydn 8% more text.txt
the quick red fox
jumped over

haydn 9%
```

whereas

```
open (WRITE, ">text.txt");
print WRITE "the lazy brown dog\n";
```

changes the file to

```
haydn 9% more text.txt
the lazy brown dog

haydn 10%
```

Note how the print statement changed. The print statement actually takes two arguments, a filehandle and the string:

```
print FILEHANDLE string
```

7.2.3 Built-in Filehandles

Perl defines several default filehandles. STDIN, STDOUT, and STDERR are connected to the Unix sources of the same name. STDIN is usually the keyboard, STDOUT and STDERR are usually the terminal. These can be changed in the Unix operating system. The print command defaults to using the STDOUT, so

```
print "mystring\n";
```

and

```
print STDOUT "mystring\n";
```

are equivalent commands.

If both STDOUT and STDERR are usually the terminal, what is the difference between them? The major difference between STDOUT and STDERR lies on the Unix command line. Unix allows you to redirect the output of a program to a file (or to another program):

```
haydn 10% test.pl > output.txt
```

The output from test.pl will now be placed into the output.txt file. However, what actually gets redirected is the STDOUT filehandle. The STDERR file handle still points to the terminal. Thus, if we wanted to print out some warning messages but not place them into the actual output, we'd write those messages to the STDERR filehandle:

```
if ($errorCondition == 3) {
  print STDERR "Warning: Non-fatal error code 3 encountered\n";
}
```

which places our warning on the screen rather than in output.txt.

It is possible to redirect the default filehandles by using them in an open statement. However, doing so isn't necessarily recommended both for practical and aesthetic reasons. However, if you have an overwhelming desire to do so, remember to preserve the original filehandles by opening them to dummy filehandles, and then restore them when you're done.

Typically, once you're done using a file you want to remember to clean up after yourself. The close() command takes care of shutting down filehandles in a consistent manner:

```
close FILEHANDLE
```

Perl will take care of shutting down filehandles when the program exits, so this step is not actually mandatory. However, shutting files after your done with them will reduce the overhead of your program and also help protect your files in the unlikely event of a water landing (or the more likely event of a system crash).

7.2.4 File Safety

Reading or writing to an undefined filehandle will at best result in an undefined value. It is usually a good idea to check and make sure the file you are attempting to open is really opened before you try to use the contents of that file. The open command returns true if it successfully opens a file, and false if you try to open a nonexistent file to read from, or if the file you want to write to cannot be opened.

Most people embed the open command in a conditional statement:

```
unless (open(INPUT, "<myfile")) {
  die "Cannot open myfile\n";
}
```

or, more commonly (and succinctly):

```
open(INPUT, "<myfile") || die "cannot open myfile\n";
```

Both pieces of code have the same effect: if the file can't be opened, the program will call the die command, which prints the warning string on STDERR. In the second form, we are again taking advantage of the shortcut evaluation of the || operator: if the file opens successfully, the left side will evaluate to true and Perl will continue on without bothering to evaluate the right side. Thus, the die command will only be evaluated if the open command fails.

Another way to check the condition of a file is to use Perl's built-in file test operators. These operators take a file name or a string and tests the file to see if a particular aspect of the file is true. The form of the file tests operators is a – followed by a character. Most operators return either true or false, but some, like the size operator, return a value. Table 7.1 summarizes some of the more commonly used file tests.

Generally, the file test operators give the programmer a finer control over the error messages and potential fixes. For example, in a program that is used by many people, we might want to check that an important file is readable by the person, and do something different if it is not:

```
unless (-r $settingFile) {
  print STDERR "Can't read settings file, using defaults\n";
  # set variables
}
```

The −r file test operators looks to see if the person who is running the program has sufficient permissions to read the file in $settingFile

Table 7.1 File test operators

operator	test
−r	file is readable
−w	file is writeable
−x	file is executable
−e	file exists
−s	file size (in bytes)
−f	file is a plain file
−d	file is a directory
−T	file is a text file
−B	file is a binary file
−M	time since last file modification (in days)
−A	time since last file access (in days)

7.2.5 The Input Operator

Once we have a filehandle to a data source, we can then use it to read or write. The Perl input operator is a filehandle flanked by the < and > symbol:

```
<FILEHANDLE>
```

The input operator reads a single line from the data source linked to the filehandle and returns TRUE if successful and FALSE otherwise. The entire line, including the "\n" is placed in the default input variable $_. Typically, the input operator is used in a while loop to read through a file line by line:

```
open (INPUT, "<sequences.fa") || die "Couldn't open file\n";
while (<INPUT>) {
  print $_;
}
close INPUT;
```

has the effect of printing out every line of the sequences.fa file onto the screen.

Using the $_ variable is handy, because it is also the default regular expression target. We don't have to do anything fancy to use a regular expression search on the input. For example, if we wanted to only print out genes identified with humans, we might write

```
open (INPUT, "<sequences.fa") || die "Couldn't open file\n";
while (<INPUT>) {
  if (/sapiens/) {print $_};
}
close INPUT;
```

The default filehandle for the input operator is STDIN. Thus

```
while (<>) { ... }
```

reads a line from STDIN, which is typically the keyboard, but can also be a Unix pipe established at the command line:

```
haydn 19% grep MDR1 sequences.fa | program.pl
```

This command runs the Unix grep command, telling it to find every line containing MDR1 in the sequences.fa file, and then sends each line to the Perl program at the other end of the pipe, where the lines can be read from the STDIN filehandle.

Even better, the Perl is smart about how it connects the STDIN and program parameters. If we try to read from STDIN, Perl looks at the parameters left in @ARGV and treats them like files to be opened for reading. For example, if program.pl contains the simple script:

```
#! /usr/bin/perl

while (<>) {
    print $_;
    $lines++;
}
print "$lines processed\n";
```

we could invoke it like so:

```
haydn 19% program.pl sequences.fa
```

and the script would proceed to print read from the file sequences.fa and print out lines.

Only parameters that remain in the @ARGV array are treated in this manner. If we have shifted a parameter out, then it is no longer available to be treated as a file. If there is more than one parameter remaining, they are all treated as files, opened sequentially for reading. So, a real example of how we might use this is a script called motifs.pl that takes a motif string and any number of sequence files:

```
#! /usr/bin/perl
# Program to scan for a motif in Fasta files

$motif = shift;

while (<>) {
    if (/$motif/) {
        print $_;
    }
}
```

The program shifts the first parameter out of the array to use as the search string, then loops through all the remaining parameters, opening the file and scanning through for the motif and printing any line that contains it. We could invoke the program like

```
% perl motif.pl ATG nr.fa rodent.fa primate.fa
```

to have Perl search the specified three files for possible start codons, or, we could rely upon the Unix wild-card expansion facility

```
% perl motif.pl ATG *.fa
```

to have Perl look through any Fasta files in our directory.

Perl is flexible about what constitutes a line of input. In actuality, Perl does not read in lines per se, but instead reads in "records." The default record separator is the newline character, "\n", which just happens to correspond to a single line of text in a file, but we can change that behavior. The chunk of text Perl treats as an input record is controlled by the special variable $/, which contains a string that is used as the input record separator. We can change $/ to suit our own needs:

```
open (INPUT, "<embl.txt") || die "Couldn't open file\n";
$/ = "||";
while (<INPUT>) {
  if (/sapiens/) {print $_};
}
close INPUT;
```

The EMBL file format separates individual records with double vertical bars (see Appendix B). By setting the $/ to "||", we effectively read the entire record, new lines and all, into the $_ variable. We can then look through the entire record to match "sapiens", which we then print out. The fact that the line returns are included in the sting actually saves us from having to worry about formatting.

Speaking of formatting, note that the input record separator is included as the last characters in the string. Often, this is inconvenient. For example, if we are reading a Fasta file into a variable in order to search it for start codons, the following simple approach of appending all the lines into a single variable won't work:

```
open (INPUT, "<seq.fa") || die "Couldn't open file\n";
while (<INPUT>) {
  $seq .= $_;
}
close INPUT;
if ($seq =~ /AUG/) {
  print "Start codon found\n";
}
```

We will miss some matches if the start codon is split across two lines, because the newline character is actually part of the string:

```
...AGGCAAGUAAGGAU\nGAAGCACUUAGGCA...
```

so we need to modify our code to remove the newlines. We can use the chomp() operator to remove the last character before we append it to our sequence string:

```
open (INPUT, "<seq.fa") || die "Couldn't open file\n";
while (<INPUT>) {
```

```
    chomp;
    $seq .= $_;
  }
  close INPUT;
  if ($seq =~ /AUG/) {
    print "Start codon found\n";
  }
```

Note that this is such a common task that the chomp operator defaults to using the $_ variable, like all other string match and manipulation commands.

The line output command is the familiar print operator. As we saw when talking about the standard filehandles, the print command actually is

```
    print FILEHANDLE string
```

The FILEHANDLE can be any filehandle that is opened appropriately for output.

7.2.6   Binary I/O

Occasionally, you might want to read from files that are not line-based text files. Certain types of data, like BLAST data files and ABI sequencer files are not text based but are actually binary files made up of 0's and 1's. As such, they don't actually have specific lines, because lines are a character-based text file nicety. Binary files also contain lots of unprintable characters. Perl provides the read() command to read binary data:

```
    read (FILEHANDLE, SCALAR, LENGTH, OFFSET)
```

Read takes LENGTH bytes of data from the FILEHANDLE and places them into SCALAR. OFFSET indicates where to begin, and the function returns the actual number of bytes read into SCALAR. A typical binary read statement would look something like

```
    $position += read(INPUT, $buffer, 256, $position)
```

and it would be embedded in a while loop that iterated over the file, doing something with the data that is placed in $buffer.

In practice, the read() command (and other associated raw binary file manipulators) should be left to people who are into pretty heavy Perl wizardry.

7.3   Interprocess Communications

Sometimes the data we want doesn't reside in a nice text file. Rather, the information is being generated by another program, and we want our program to extract the information on the fly. Perl provides several good resources for getting information on the fly from active sources.

7.3.1   Processes

In computer parlance, when a program has loaded code into memory and is executing it becomes known as a process (or, alternately, as a thread). In modern computers, several processes can be (and usually are) running at the same time. Under the Unix operating system, you can get a list of active processes using the ps command:

```
haydn 3% ps -ef
UID            PID   PPID  C    STIME TTY       TIME CMD
cjamison      8022   8007  0 00:47:38 ?        0:10 netscape
cjamison      3822   3775  0   Aug 06 pts/0   14:01 xemacs
cjamison      8084   8059  0 00:17:58 pts/1    0:00 -tcsh
cjamison      8213   8209  0 03:31:17 pts/2    0:00 -tcsh
cjamison      8227   8213  0 03:31:34 pts/2    0:00 ps -ef
```

The partial listing of processes running on my machine shows that there were two command shells (tcsh), one copy of xemacs, and one copy of netscape. At any one time, there can be hundreds of processes running on a moderately busy computer.

   The computer keeps track of processes by their process ID (PID), which is a unique number attached to the process when it is created. In a true multiprocess environment, processes can create other processes in a procedure called spawning. When a process spawns a new process, the original process is called the parent and the new one is called the child. Child processes usually keep track of their parent processes so they can report back. In the list above, the ps command has a PID of 8227, and a parent PPID of 8213. Looking back up the list, we see that one of the tcsh shells has a PID of 8213, showing that the ps process was spawned by that shell.

7.3.2   Process Pipes

The most common use of process pipes is to get information from a system command. For example, we might want to get a list of all the files in the current directory. For this, we can simply use the backtick (or grave accent) quotation marks to interpolate our string into a system command like we saw in Chapter 2. We can take the output and assign it to a variable:

```
$dir = 'ls -lag';
print $dir;
```

This code will store the entire output from the ls command into the $dir variable, which we then print out:

```
drwxrwxrwx  28 cjamison staff   908 May 26 13:08 .
drwxrwxrwx  20 cjamison staff   636 May 19 12:17 ..
-rw-r--r--   1 cjamison staff   119 May 19 13:56 genes.txt
-rw-r--r--   1 cjamison staff   123 May 19 16:56 hello.pl
```

```
-rw-r--r--   1 cjamison staff   127 May 19 16:52 hello.pl~
-rw-r--r--   1 cjamison staff   446 May 25 18:24 mop.pl
-rw-r--r--   1 cjamison staff   447 May 25 18:23 mop.pl~
-rw-r--r--   1 cjamison staff   227 May 24 17:36 refsub.pl
-rw-r--r--   1 cjamison staff   185 May 24 17:33 refsub.pl~
-rw-r--r--   1 cjamison staff   123 May 19 16:56 trash.txt
```

Getting results from the system via the interpolation of a command string is straightforward, but limited. For example, we might be interested only in the Perl scripts that have a.pl extension, and so we would want to filter the output of the ls command line-by-line.

A special type of Perl file handle exists to communicate with the computer operating system. These are commonly called pipes, because they pipe data from one process to another. Typically in Perl programs, the item on the other end of the pipe is a system command that we want to get information either to or from, so rather than giving the open() command a file name, we give it a system command. We use the | symbol to tell Perl the filehandle is a pipe, and we differentiate which direction the data is flowing by at which end of the system command we place it. If we place the | in front of the command, data flows from Perl to the command, whereas if we place it at the end, data flows from the command to Perl. Thus

```
open (DIR, "ls -lag|");
while (<DIR>) {
  if (/\.pl$/) {
     print $_;
  }
}
```

creates a pipe with data flowing from the ls command into Perl. The while loop then reads from the pipe, checking to see if the line we just read contains the.pl extension at the end of the line before printing the file name. The output

```
-rw-r--r--   1 cjamison staff   123 May 19 16:56 hello.pl
-rw-r--r--   1 cjamison staff   446 May 25 18:24 mop.pl
-rw-r--r--   1 cjamison staff   227 May 24 17:36 refsub.pl
```

shows that indeed we have now filtered our ls command to list only the Perl scripts in the directory.

We can read and write to pipes just like any other filehandle, bearing in mind that there is an active program at the other end of the pipe, and the response of the program is sensitive to how fast the program runs.

7.3.3 Creating Processes

Perl allows us to create child processes within our program. We do this when we need to have an autonomous process occurring outside the main process, like when we want to wait for input, or to repeat a loop until interrupted by a keystroke. The command we use is the fork() command. The fork() command creates a second process, loading in a second copy of the code to serve as the child. Execution of the code in both processes continues from the statement that contained the fork() command.

We can tell the difference between the parent and the child process by the value returned by the fork() command. In the parent process, fork returns the PID of the child, while to the child it returns a 0 (if the fork fails, the command returns a undefined value). The value returned is usually used to determine what code is executed by the two processes.

```
$pid = fork;
if ($pid) {
  # parent code goes here
  # child PID is in $pid
} elsif ($pid == 0) {
  #child code goes here
  exit;
} else {
  die "fork failed.";
}
```

The fork code is actually quite simple. First, we execute the fork, storing the return value in $pid, and then we use that value to conditionally control the execution. If the value is a number (thus registering as TRUE in a Boolean context), we know that this is the parent process. If the value is equal to 0, we know that we are in the child process. If the value is undefined, we have encountered some sort of error. Note that we explicitly placed an exit command at the end of the child code. This is to prevent the child from continuing on and executing any parental code that follows the conditional.

7.3.4 Monitoring Processes

The parent can use the PID returned from fork to monitor the child process. The child process (or any Perl program) can get the parent PID using the getppid() command. We can use the PIDs to control the timing of our processes. For example, our parent process might need to make sure the child has finished before proceeding. For this we can use the wait commands. There are two different commands:

```
wait
waitpid(PID, FLAGS)
```

Both commands do similar things: they wait until a process is finished before allowing the program to continue. The wait() command simply stops the program until a child process dies, then returns the PID of the deceased process. But because the wait() command doesn't care exactly which child process has died, it is safer to use the waitpid() command that monitors a specific PID, and returns true when the process dies. Both commands return a −1 if there are no child processes.

Both wait() and waitpid() wait an unspecified amount of time, which is fine if your child process is unlikely to hang. But if there is a chance for an infinite loop, or if you want to simply keep track of a process for a specified time period, then waiting for a process to exit itself is insufficient. The kill() command allows you to execute processes that have gone on too long.

```
kill (SIGNAL, PID_LIST)
```

The signals for the Perl kill() command are the same as those for the Unix kill command (see the man page for kill), and can either be the integer or the string representation. The PID_LIST is a list of valid PIDs to kill. So, if we wanted our child process to run exactly five minutes, we could write

```
if ($pid = fork) {
  sleep 300;
  kill (9, $pid);
} else {
  ## do something for about five minutes
}
```

7.3.5 Implicit Forks

Some Perl commands perform an implicit fork, spawning their own processes and then waiting for the response. We have already seen an example of this when we opened a filehandle as a pipe:

```
open(GREP, "grep MDR1 fastalib|");
while (<GREP>) {
  if (/human/i) {
      print $_ . "\n";
  }
}
close GREP;
```

In this case, a child process was created and associated with the GREP filehandle using the open() command. We read lines from that filehandle, printing out any that contain the word human, until the GREP filehandle indicates it is done, then we use the close() command to clean up the filehandle. The close() command is always polite: it will wait until the process attached to pipe indicates it is finished before it closes the filehandle.

In the GREP example we were running another program on the computer. We can accomplish a similar task using the system() command:

```
system "cp library.fa library.back";
```

We use the system() command if we don't care so much about getting the output of the program, because there is no connection between the process and the Perl I/O filehandles. Like the open() command, the system() performs an implicit fork and waits for the program to finish.

Finally, we can get the program output back as a string if we use the back tick operators:

```
$lines = 'grep mouse fastalib';
```

places the output from the grep program into $lines. The back tick operators also allow for variable interpolation, so we can write:

```
$lines = 'grep $keyword fastalib';
```

Chapter Summary

- Program parameters typed on the command line can be read from the @ARGV array.

- A filehandle is a data structure that names an input or output pipe.

- STDIN is the default input filehandle.

- STDOUT and STDERR are the default output filehandles.

- A filehandle can be attached to a file using the open() command.

- A filehandle is detached from a file using the close() command.

- The input operator <> reads from STDIN (or a specified filehandle) and puts the input record into the $_ variable.

- Process pipes, back tick quotes, and the system function allow Perl programs to communicate to programs

For More Information

```
perldoc perlopentut
```

Exercises

1. Define the term I/O pipe.

2. What is the relationship of STDIN, STDOUT, and STDERR to the normal Unix input and output devices?

3. How can you ensure that the user supplied the proper number of parameters?

Programming Challenges

1. Write a program that reads in a text file and prints out the first 20 lines to the screen. (*Hint*: You will need to use @ARGV to get the file name). For extra credit, make your program accept any number of file names and iterate through them.

2. Write a program that reads a GenBank file from disk and outputs a Fasta formatted file (see Appendix B for file formats).

Chapter 8

Perl Modules and Packages

As we write more and more programs, we often find ourselves using the same subroutines over and over. For example, a program to predict primer pairs and a program to look for open reading frames both need a subroutine to reverse complement the input file. It would be nice to be able to have a generic library code that we can include in our programs, so all that we have to do is to call the subroutine and not have to worry about copying the subroutine from one program to another.

8.1 Modules

Fortunately, Perl has just exactly that mechanism. A Perl module is simply a text file containing Perl code. The file is placed in a special directory, and then named with a .pm extension. Code from the module can be brought into the current program with the use statement:

```
use module_dir::module;
```

and instantly all the code within the module is available for use. This includes any variables and subroutines written there.

So, suppose we wanted to create a Perl module that contained some useful sequence manipulation subroutines. We would create a file called "SequenceRoutines.pm" and put our subroutines into it. For now, we have two:

Perl Programming for Biologists, D. Curtis Jamison
ISBN 0-471-43059-5 Copyright © 2003 Wiley-Liss, Inc.

```
# generate a random DNA sequence
sub RandomSeq {
  @nucleotides = ('a','c','g','t');
  my $length = shift || 40;
  my $retval = "";
  for (my $i = 0; $i < $length; $i++) {
      my $base = $nucleotides[int(rand(4))];
      $retval .= $base;
  }
  return $retval;
}

# reverse complement a DNA sequence
sub ReverseComplement {
  my $seq = shift;
  my $retval = reverse($seq);
  $retval ~= tr/actg/tgac/g;
  return $retval;
}

1
```

Note the bare 1 at the end of the file. This is not a misprint. The use command looks at the last line in the module for a TRUE value, which indicates that the module loaded correctly. The bare 1 signals the use command that it has indeed reached the end of the module and can proceed with the program.

After we have created the file, we either have to put it into the proper directory for Perl, or we have to tell Perl how to find it. It is useful to know where Perl is looking for modules, which we can find out using the −V switch. Simply type

```
% perl −V
```

and Perl responds with a description of how it is configured. At or near the end, there is a line that says @INC and is followed by a list of directory paths:

```
@INC:
    /System/Library/Perl/darwin
    /System/Library/Perl
    /Library/Perl/darwin
    /Library/Perl
    /Library/Perl
    /Network/Library/Perl/darwin
    /Network/Library/Perl
    /Network/Library/Perl
```

is what it looks like under Mac OS X. The @INC list is all the directories where Perl is looking for modules. If you have sufficient user privileges, you can put your Perl module in one of these directories. However, most of us don't have permission, so we have to figure out another way to deal with it.

First, note that the . directory is part of the directory list. The . directory is simply Unix shorthand for the current directory. So your programs will always look in the current directory for .pm files. However, that creates a problem if you try to run a program that uses a .pm file from another directory. The easiest way to deal with the problem is to simply put our .pm file into a logical place, and then push the new path onto the @INC array:

```
push (@INC, "/usr/home/cjamison/perlib");
```

tells Perl to look in my perlib directory for any modules it can't find elsewhere.

Now we can utilize the subroutines in the SequenceRoutines.pm file simply by including the file in our program:

```
push (@INC, "/usr/home/cjamison/perlib");

use SequenceRoutines;
$forward = RandomSeq(80);
$reverse = ReverseComplement($forward);
```

After the use statement, the two subroutines in SequenceRoutine.pm are available to our program exactly as if they had been written in the same file. For simple libraries this is fine. However, there are situations that can create complications.

The primary complication is the potential for two subroutines that share a name. For example, consider a situation where we've been using the SequenceRoutines.pm library for a while in various programs, and we decide that the library module really needs to have GCContent() routine, since we've written it for four or five of our programs. So we create the routine in SequenceRoutines.pm. But now, the previous programs where we have written a GCContent() subroutine have two identically named subroutines: one that was written in the main program file, and one that was included by the use command. When GCContent() is used, there is no guarantee which version we will get. Fortunately, Perl has a way around this problem, but to use it effectively we need a little background first.

8.2 Packages

In Chapter 1, we learned that when the interpreter starts up, it sets aside a table in memory that keeps track of the names of all the variables and subroutines. This table is called the name table, and all the entries within the name table constitute the namespace of the program. When a new variable or a new subroutine is created, the name is placed into the name table with a pointer to the memory location where the value or the code is stored. If the name has been seen before, Perl fetches the value out of the memory location, or stores a new value in the memory location.

Perl allows us to create and use multiple namespaces. The package command switches between namespaces, creating new ones as required. The syntax is

```
package mypackage;
```

and all variables and subroutines that appear after the package name are in the mypackage namespace.

As a simple example, consider the ReverseComplement() subroutine. The code works well for DNA, but we might want a version that works with RNA. One way to do this is to create separate namespaces for DNA and RNA, each with a ReverseComplement() subroutine:

```perl
package DNA_Utilities;

# DNA nucleotides
@nucleotides = ('a', 'c', 't', 'g');

sub ReverseComplement {
  my $seq = shift;
  my $retval = reverse($seq);
  $retval ~= tr/actg/tgac/g;
  return $retval;
}

package RNA_Utilities;

#RNA nucleotides
@nucleotides = ('a', 'c', 'u', 'g');

sub ReverseComplement {
  my $seq = shift;
  my $retval = reverse($seq);
  $retval ~= tr/acug/ugac/g;
  return $retval;
}

1;
```

When this code is executed, Perl creates a namespace called "DNA_Utilities" and puts an array called "nucleotides" and a subroutine called "ReverseComplement" into it. At the second package command, Perl creates another namespace called "RNA_Utilities" and places an array called "nucleotides" and a subroutine called "ReverseComplement" into it. Even though they have similar names, the two arrays and two subroutines are distinct and different because they are in different namespaces. We can use either version of ReverseComplement() simply by the use of qualified names, which simply means we join the namespace to the front of the name with a pair of colons. Thus we can write:

```perl
$DNA_Seq = "AATGAATGGCTAGCTTAGGCTAGGTTCCCATGATGG";
$RNA_Seq = "AAUGAAUGGCUAGCUUAGGCUAGGUUCCCAUGAUGG";
$DNA_RevSeq = DNA_Utilities::ReverseComplement($DNA_Seq);
$RNA_RevSeq = RNA_Utilities::ReverseComplement($RNA_Seq);
```

which is a completely distinctive way to access the subroutines.

Because ReverseComplement() is a subroutine, we don't use a variable prefix when we refer to it. But we still need to use them for ordinary variables. Because the namespace is a qualifier for the name, the variable prefix still goes in the very front. So, to use the arrays, we would write

```
print (@DNA_Utilities::nucleotides);
```

or

```
print (@RNA_Utilities::nucleotides);
```

8.3   Combining Packages and Modules

Typically, packages have a one-to-one relationship with modules. That is, packages are organized into modules with one package per module. Almost every Perl module begins with a package command, so when we include a module with the use statement we are creating a new namespace.

To make our life easier (and to help prevent collisions), the convention is to name the package and module with the same name. Thus, for our original utility module, because we stored it in the SequenceRoutines.pm module, we would create a namespace called SequenceRoutines:

```
package SequenceRoutines;
@nucleotides = ('a','c','g','t');

sub RandomSeq {
  my $length = shift || 40;
  my $retval = "";
  for (my $i = 0; $i < $length; $i++) {
     my $base = $nucleotides[int(rand(4))];
     $retval .= $base;
  }
  return $retval;
}

sub ReverseComplement {
  my $seq = shift;
  my $retval = reverse($seq);
  $retval ~= tr/actg/tgac/g;
  return $retval;
}

1
```

and to use it our programs would look like

```
use SequenceRoutines;
$forward = SequenceRoutines::RandomSeq(80);
$reverse = SequenceRoutines::ReverseComplement($forward);
```

Although a bit wordier, it is much clearer where the subroutines are coming from without any ambiguity about what namespace they are using.

8.4   Included Modules

Several incredibly useful modules are already included in the standard Perl distribution. These modules are ones that proved to be so wildly popular that everyone was downloading and installing them. So to save wear and tear on the CPAN servers, these modules are included right from the start.

8.4.1   CGI

Perl is often used to write scripts that process hypertext forms on the WWW. These scripts make use of a protocol called the Common Gateway Interface, or CGI. The CGI.pm module by Lincoln Stein makes it easy to both programmatically create and parse HTML fill-out forms.

CGI.pm contains methods that provide shortcuts to produce HTML pages that range from simple static displays to complex forms with cookies, style sheets, and frames. Additionally, the module has methods for retrieving data from forms and populating Perl variables with the data.

8.4.2   Getopt

The usual method of passing arguments to Perl programs as a list of strings on the command line is fine for most programs. However, we often find that the simple protocol becomes inadequate. For example, consider a program that will take accession numbers from different databases and fetch the sequence record. How can we programmatically tell which database the accession numbers belong to?

One method might be to require the user to type in the name of the database as an argument:

```
haydn%>getSequence.pl GenBank AC000123
```

We can achieve the same effect without a lot of extra typing by implementing single-character switches

```
haydn%>getSequence.pl -G AC000123
```

Switches can also serve as Boolean markers to control our program. We can improve our getSequence.pl script by adding the ability to reverse complement the sequence if we see the – R switch. So, in our hypothetical program, typing

```
haydn%>getSequence.pl -G AC000123 -R
```

will return the reverse complement of our sequence.

Regular Unix commands also use switches (*e.g.*, ls -lag), so our getSequence.pl program will look a lot like other commands. But we do have to be careful, because in Unix the order of the switches doesn't matter, so we have to be able to process

```
haydn%>getSequence.pl -R -G AC000123
```

as well as

```
haydn%>getSequence.pl -RG AC000123
```

the latter being an example of switch clustering. Clearly, performing this task will take fancy processing of the @ARGV array.

Fortunately, the Getopt distribution makes dealing with command line switches straightforward. You simply tell Getopt what switches to look for, and the subroutine will parse @ARGV removing any switches and setting variables.

Getopt consists of two modules: Long.pm and Std.pm. The Std.pm module is simpler and will take care of 90% of your needs. Std.pm contains the getopts() command, which takes a string that tells it which single characters to look for as switches. A character followed by a colon means that there is an argument to go with the switch. For each switch it finds, the getopts() command sets the variable $opt_*, where the * is replaced by the switch, and the value of the $opt_* variable is either 1 or is the value passed.

Thus, to implement our example, we simply write a main code that looks like

```
#!/usr/local/bin/perl

use Getopts::Std;
use SequenceRoutines;

getopts('RG:S:P');
if ($opt_G) {
  $seq = getGenBank($opt_G);
}
elsif ($opt_S) {
  $seq = getSwissProt($opt_S);
}
elsif ($opt_P) {
  $seq = getPBD($opt_P);
}

if ($opt_R) {
  reverseComplement($seq);
}
```

The program consists of a series of tests to see if a particular $opt_* variable is set, and, if it is, we perform whatever task is controlled by that variable, either retrieving a sequence from the database or reverse complementing the sequence. Note the actual subroutines for fetching the sequence have been left out of the example, but we would probably use the BioPerl database routines.

8.4.3 IO

There are six modules that are part of the IO package: IO::Handle, IO::Seekable, IO::File, IO::Pipe, IO::Socket, and IO::Dir. Each of these modules provides an object-oriented interface to the Perl IO routines. Although not overly useful for small scripts, these modules are invaluable when writing larger object-oriented programs, because they help create an object orientation for our entire program.

8.4.4 File::Path

The File::Path module provides an easy way to create and manage directories from within a Perl program. For example, seqfiles.pl is a script for a sequencing project that automatically creates a directory structure for use with the phred, phrap, and consed programs and transfers the sequencer files into it. To do this, we use the mkpath subroutine:

```
#! /usr/bin/perl

# Move sequence files to a specific directory

use File::Path;

$basedir = '/local/data/sequencing/';
$project = shift;
$filedir = shift;

$chromat_dir = $basedir . $project . "/chromat_dir";
$edit_dir = $basedir . $project . "/edit_dir";

mkpath($chromat_dir);
mkpath($edit_dir);

system "mv $filedir/\* $chromat_dir";
```

The script first brings in the File::Path module, which gives us access to the mkpath subroutine. Then it sets an absolute path to the standard sequence data directory, gets the project name, and gets the directory name for the chromatographs. Then it builds the necessary file names for the phred/phrap programs by concatenating the base directory name, the project name, and the name of the required phred/phrap directories. Next it creates the directories using the mkpath subroutine, and then it moves the files into the appropriate directory using the system command. We invoke the script like

```
%seqfiles.pl MDR /local/incoming
```

and moments later all the files that were in /local/incoming are moved to /local/data/sequencing/MDR/chromat_dir.

The mkpath routine will create all the needed directories leading up to and including the specified one. Thus if /local/data/sequencing didn't exist, the mkpath subroutine would create it. The subroutine returns a list of all the directories it creates.

3.4.5 Strict

The strict module is used to check your code to make sure that you have not accidentally used unsafe constructs. For example, strict makes sure that all variables are either scoped using the my command or use fully qualified names. The use of a global variable causes the script to fail.

Currently, the module will enforce rules about variables, references, and subroutines. You simply put

```
use strict;
```

at the beginning of your program and Perl will force you to write perfect code.

Often, the strict module is too strict. For example, the code in seqfiles.pl would cause strict to be upset about the fact that none of the variables were scoped with the my command. However, because the script is so small and simple there really wasn't a big need to be strict about global variables. So, when you include the strict module, you can tell it what you want to be strict about. You simply include a string with the use command:

```
use strict "subs";
```

which causes the module to be strict only about how we use subroutines. Similarly, "vars" makes strict worry only about variables, and "refs" makes it worry only about references.

Another way to deal with strict is to specifically turn one aspect of strict off with the "no strict" command. For example, in seqfiles.pl we might want to only turn off the variable checking, so we would rewrite our code to look like:

```
#! /usr/bin/perl

# Move sequence files to a specific directory

use strict;
no strict "vars";
use File::Path;

$basedir = '/local/data/sequencing/';
$project = shift;
$filedir = shift;

$chromat_dir = $basedir . $project . "/chromat_dir";
$edit_dir = $basedir . $project . "/edit_dir";

mkpath($chromat_dir);
mkpath($edit_dir);

system "mv $filedir/\* $chromat_dir";
```

Now the program will run just fine with the global variables, while still being strict about the references and the subroutines.

In general, if you are writing a large Perl program with many subroutines and modules, it is a good idea to use strict.

8.5   The CPAN

The included modules barely scratch the surface of available modules. Literally hundreds of useful modules are available to Perl programmers. The problem comes from knowing where to find information about available modules, and which ones to choose.

Fortunately, we don't have to hunt all over the Web to find modules. Most are collected for us in the CPAN: the Comprehensive Perl Archive Network. We can connect to the CPAN at http://www.cpan.org and either browse or search through all the contributed modules there. Then, if we like it, we can download a module and install it in our Perl modules directory. Most modules come with a very detailed set of instructions on how to install them.

Although browsing the CPAN using a Web browser is straightforward, the standard Perl distribution contains a module that makes life much easier. The CPAN.pm module allows us to download and install new modules. Additionally, we can use CPAN.pm to manage our installed modules (*i.e.*, if we're fortunate enough to have a Unix computer, as CPAN.pm doesn't work under Windows or MacOS 9).

8.5.1   Setting Up the CPAN Module

Because CPAN.pm is part of the standard Perl distribution, we can simply begin using it. To launch the interactive CPAN shell, we run Perl in the interactive mode, using the -M switch to load the CPAN module and the -e switch to run the shell subroutine:

```
[haydn:~] cjamison% perl -MCPAN -e shell

cpan shell -- CPAN exploration and modules installation (v1.52)

cpan>
```

The CPAN shell is now running. If you have never run the CPAN before, the shell program will create a .cpan subdirectory in your home directory, and then try to configure the setting needed to successfully use the program. The first question CPAN asks you is:

```
Are you ready for manual configuration? [yes]
```

If you desire, you can answer "no" to this question, in which case the script will attempt to automatically figure out the configuration. However, the autoconfig function is less than perfect, and it typically fails to fully configure properly (often failing to find key programs that really are present). It is better to answer "yes" and run the configuration program manually.

For each configuration question, the script makes a best guess and places it in square brackets at the end of the question. This is the default value, which you can accept simply by hitting return. If the default value is wrong, or if you just want to change it, you simply type in the new value. For example, the config script asks for the location of certain important programs:

```
Where is your gzip program? [/usr/bin/gzip]
Where is your tar program? [/usr/bin/tar]
Warning: unzip not found in PATH
Where is your unzip program? [] /usr/bin/gunzip
Warning: make not found in PATH
Where is your make program? [] /usr/sbin/make
```

The first two needed programs, gzip and tar, were found by the script with no problem. Hitting return sufficed to enter these two programs into the configuration file. However, the unzip and make programs weren't found, so the default was left blank and I had to type in the values (a nonstandard unzip program and a make program in an odd place found through the which command). Obviously, you need to be relatively familiar with your Unix system when running the config script.

The config also asks you to choose one or more CPAN FTP mirror sites. The CPAN module will download a list of CPAN mirror sites and shows them to you in a numbered list. Choose a few sites that are relatively close and type the numbers one at a time at the prompt. When you have entered several, hit return without entering a number and the script will proceed.

During the course of the installation, the CPAN script will make a few suggestions to you about upgrading your installation. These are typically good suggestions to follow. Make a note of the suggestions as they come up, and install the recommended upgrades when possible.

After the installation script is finished, it will commit the configuration to a special file called MyConfig.pm, which is buried deep in your .cpan directory. This file will be loaded from now on whenever you run the CPAN module, and the install script won't run again. You now should be at the cpan> prompt.

8.5.2   Finding Modules

The most important command to remember when running the CPAN shell interactively is the ? command. Typing the question mark at the cpan> prompt will cause a detailed help screen to show up:

```
cpan> ?

Display Information
 a                                          authors
 b              string           display    bundles
 d              or               info       distributions
 m              /regex/          about      modules
 i              or                          anything of above
 r              none             reinstall  recommendations
 u                               uninstalled distributions

Download, Test, Make, Install...
 get                             download
 make                            make (implies get)
 test           modules,         make test (implies make)
 install        dists, bundles   make install (implies test)
 clean                           make clean
 look                            open subshell in these dists'
directories
 readme                          display these dists' README
files

Other
 h,?            display this menu      ! perl-code    eval a
perl command
 o conf [opt]   set and query options  q             quit
the cpan shell
 reload cpan    load CPAN.pm again      reload index  load
newer indices
 autobundle     Snapshot                force cmd
unconditionally do cmd
cpan>
```

This screen lists all the commands that the CPAN shell script understands. The commands fall into three general categories: information, installation, and management. We will consider each set of commands in turn.

The information commands allow you to search out modules based upon things like the author's name or the name of the module. The information commands will accept either a string or a regular expression.

We can find out information about bundles, distributions, and modules using the b, d, and m commands, respectively. Bundles are sets of modules that are required for the proper installation and running of a particular module. For example,

```
cpan> b BioPerl

Trying with "/usr/bin/ncftp -c" to get

ftp://ftp.perl.org/pub/CPAN/authors/id/C/CR/CRAFFI/Bundle-BioPerl-
    1.00.tar.gz
```

```
Bundle-BioPerl-1.00
Bundle-BioPerl-1.00/BioPerl.pm
Bundle-BioPerl-1.00/Makefile.PL
Bundle-BioPerl-1.00/Changes
Bundle-BioPerl-1.00/README
Bundle-BioPerl-1.00/MANIFEST
Bundle id = Bundle::BioPerl
    CPAN_USERID  CRAFFI (Chris Dagdigian <dag@sonsorol.org>)
    CPAN_VERSION 1.00
    CPAN_FILE    C/CR/CRAFFI/Bundle-BioPerl-1.00.tar.gz
    MANPAGE      Bundle::BioPerl - A bundle to install
external CPAN modules used by BioPerl
    CONTAINS     Bundle::LWP, File::Temp, IO::Scalar,
IO::String, HTTP::Request::Common, HTTP::Status,
LWP::UserAgent, URI::Escape, XML::Parser,
XML::Parser::PerlSAX, XML::Writer, XML::Node
    INST_FILE    /Users/cjamison/.cpan/Bundle/BioPerl.pm
    INST_VERSION 1.00

cpan>
```

is a list of modules required for BioPerl.

Distributions are a complete set of related modules. For example, the CGI distribution is made up of six modules, as seen in the information query:

```
cpan> d /CGI.pm-2.80/
Distribution id = L/LD/LDS/CGI.pm-2.80.tar.gz
    CONTAINSMODS CGI::Carp CGI::Fast CGI::Cookie CGI::Push
       CGI::Util CGI
    CPAN_USERID  LDS (Lincoln D. Stein <lstein@cshl.org>)

cpan>
```

The i command looks for any information it can find about the search string. It will bring back a list of all authors, bundles, distributions, and modules that match the string. Once you find the items you are interested in, you can get more information about them using the a, b, d, or m command. Be prepared for some rather long lists though: if your search term is too generic, you can get back several screens worth of listing.

When you first run an information request, the CPAN shell goes out to the CPAN site you specified and fetches back several index files, which it places in your.cpan directory. All searches are run against the local copy of the index files unless you request information from a file that has not yet been cached. If you suspect that something has changed since you last connected, you can use the reload command, which forces the CPAN shell to go out and refresh the cache files.

3.5.3 Installing Modules

The installation commands in the CPAN shell are extremely straightforward. All of the commands work with modules, distributions, or bundles. Although all the commands accept either strings or regular expressions, it is better to use the full string name to avoid any confusion of multiple modules.

The get command goes out and fetches items from the CPAN mirror you specified. The make command runs commands to create the Perl module, compiling any special external programs required. The test command will run a script supplied with the module that checks the functionality of the module to make sure it was created properly. Finally, the install command places the new module(s) into the proper Perl directory.

These four commands form a nice flow: To have a working Perl module you must first get it, then make it, test it, and finally install it. Moreover, you can't take these steps out of order. You must first get a module before you can make it. So the CPAN shell assumes that the act of issuing the commands for the later steps implies that you want to perform the earlier steps. Thus, if you want to install a newer version of the CGI module, you simply ask the CPAN shell to install it and everything flows from there:

```
cpan> install CGI
Running install for module CGI
Running make for L/LD/LDS/CGI.pm-2.80.tar.gz
Fetching with LWP:

ftp://ftp.dc.aleron.net/pub/CPAN/authors/id/L/LD/LDS/CGI.pm-
   2.80.tar.gz
CPAN: MD5 loaded ok
Fetching with LWP:

ftp://ftp.dc.aleron.net/pub/CPAN/authors/id/L/LD/LDS/CHECKSUMS
Checksum for
/usr/local/lib/perl5/CPAN/sources/authors/id/L/LD/LDS/CGI.pm-
   2.80.tar.gz
ok
Scanning cache /usr/local/lib/perl5/CPAN/build for sizes
x CGI.pm-2.80/t/lib/Test/Simple.pm, 12739 bytes, 25 blocks
...
x CGI.pm-2.80/cgi-lib_porting.html, 8714 bytes, 18 blocks

   CPAN.pm: Going to build L/LD/LDS/CGI.pm-2.80.tar.gz

Checking if your kit is complete...
Looks good
Writing Makefile for CGI
cp CGI/Push.pm blib/lib/CGI/Push.pm
...
cp CGI.pm blib/lib/CGI.pm
   /sbin/make  -- OK
Running make test
        PERL_DL_NONLAZY =1 /usr/bin/perl -Iblib/arch -Iblib/lib
-I/usr/local/lib/perl5/5.6.1/IP30-irix
   -I/usr/local/lib/perl5/5.6.1
-e 'use Test::Harness qw(&runtests $verbose); $verbose =0;
   runtests
```

```
@ARGV;' t/*.t
t/apache...........ok
...
t/util.............ok
All tests successful, 8 subtests skipped.
Files =12, Tests =315,  6 wallclock secs ( 4.36 cusr +  0.60 csys
  =  4.96 CPU)
  /sbin/make test -- OK
Running make install
Installing /usr/local/lib/perl5/5.6.1/CGI.pm
...
Installing /usr/local/lib/perl5/5.6.1/CGI/Cookie.pm
Writing /usr/local/lib/perl5/5.6.1/IP30-irix/auto/CGI/.packlist
Appending installation info to
/usr/local/lib/perl5/5.6.1/IP30-irix/perllocal.pod
  /sbin/make install  -- OK

cpan>
```

Because install implies test and test implies make, the CPAN shell first tries to make the CGI programs. But make implies get, so before going on with the make program the CPAN shell issues the command to get the CGI distribution we specified. After the get command successfully fetches the file, the make command resumes. When the make command successfully finishes, the test command takes over. When the test command finishes, we now have returned to the install command, and the install command places the CGI.pm modules into our module directory.

The clean command will take care of removing the old distributions files. Once you have installed a module or distribution, you can save a lot of disk space by wiping out all the intermediate files.

```
cpan> clean B/BI/BIRNEY/bioperl-0.05.1.tar.gz
Running make clean
```

The install commands work with your local module directory. Perl doesn't really care where modules are stored, so you can put them locally in your own directory and use them in your script from there via the @INC list. However, this has the effect of hard-coding your specific module path into your script, thereby reducing the portability.

Often it is better to install the modules into the main Perl module directory. This has the advantage that the modules are globally available and you no longer have to worry about altering the @INC list. The downside is that if you don't have the proper access permissions, you will have to bribe the system administrator to install the packages you want (fortunately, system administrators have a notorious weakness for chocolate chip cookies).

8.5.4 Managing Installed Modules

The r command asks the CPAN script to look through your installed packages and make recommendations about modules that might need to be updated. The list that is returned contains the name of the module, the version installed on your computer, and the latest version in the CPAN:

```
cpan> r

Package namespace          installed    latest   in CPAN file
AutoLoader                      5.57      5.58
    G/GS/GSAR/perl-5.6.1.tar.gz
CGI                             2.56      2.80
    L/LD/LDS/CGI.pm-2.80.tar.gz
CGI::Pretty                     1.03      1.05
    L/LD/LDS/CGI.pm-2.77.tar.gz
CPAN                            1.52      1.59
    A/AN/ANDK/CPAN-1.59.tar.gz
DB_File                         1.72      1.802
    P/PM/PMQS/DB_File-1.802.tar.gz
ExtUtils::Embed                 1.01      1.2505
    D/DO/DOUGM/ExtUtils-Embed-1.14.tar.gz
File::Spec                       0.8      0.82
    R/RB/RBS/File-Spec-0.82.tar.gz
Getopt::Long                    2.23      2.26
    J/JV/JV/Getopt-Long-2.26.tar.gz
Math::BigFloat                 undef      1.27
    T/TE/TELS/Math-BigInt-1.49.tar.gz
Net::Ping                       2.02      2.11
    B/BB/BBB/Net-Ping-2.11.tar.gz
Pod::Checker                   1.098      1.2
    B/BR/BRADAPP/PodParser-1.18.tar.gz
Pod::Man                        1.02      1.32
    R/RR/RRA/podlators-1.20.tar.gz
Term::Cap                      undef      1.07
    J/JS/JSTOWE/Term-Cap-1.07.tar.gz
Test                            1.13      1.20
    M/MS/MSCHWERN/Test-1.20.tar.gz
Test::Harness                 1.1604      2.01
    M/MS/MSCHWERN/Test-Harness-2.01.tar.gz
Text::Soundex                    1.0      2.20
    M/MA/MARKM/Text-Soundex-2.20.tar.gz
Text::Wrap                  98.11290   2001.092
    M/MU/MUIR/modules/Text-Tabs+Wrap-2001.0929.tar.gz
1 installed module has a version number of 0
84 installed modules have no parseable version number

cpan>
```

Based upon this list, it looks like the Perl installation on my laptop needs quite a bit of maintenance. On the other hand, many of the outdated packages aren't too troubling (like Net::Ping) and with others I'm happy with the version that is installed (like CGI and DB_File) because they're working fine and the newer versions don't contain any must-have features. Ultimately, you will have to decide which modules are the most important and useful for your own tasks.

There are a couple caveats about using the r command. First, the modules that are out of date are often in the original Perl distribution. Without having root permission, you can't update those packages. Second, you should be aware that updated packages can be incompatible with earlier versions. If you follow good object-oriented Perl programming techniques, your scripts should be relatively insulated from changes in the inner workings of modules, but be aware that reinstalling a newer version of a module might break an older piece of code. Finally, be aware that updating some modules might trigger a reinstall of Perl itself! The best advice when using the CPAN is to be conservative.

Chapter Summary

- Perl modules are reusable code libraries.

- Modules are included into a program with the use() command.

- Module files must end with a positive statement (usually a bare 1).

- Packages keep the namespaces straight.

- The package() command creates a new namespace.

- Fully qualified names consist of the package name and the variable or subroutine name concatenated with a pair of colons.

- Packages typically have a one-to-one relationship with modules.

- Modules already exist for many common Perl programming tasks.

- Some modules come preinstalled. Other modules can be fetched from the CPAN.

For More Information

```
perldoc perlmod
perldoc perlmodlib
perldoc CGI.pm
perldoc Getopt/Std.pm
perldoc CPAN.pm
www.cpan.org
```

Exercises

1. What is the difference between a module and a package?

2. Make a list of other routines might be useful in SequenceRoutines.

3. How many packages can exist in a program?

4. Explain what is meant by a fully qualified name.

5. What modules are included in your Perl installation?

6. Use the CPAN to answer the following:

    a. What is the latest version of BioPerl?

    b. Who is the author of GetOpts?

    c. How many modules have the word "math" in their name?

    d. How up to date is your Perl installation?

7. Explain the difference between a module and a bundle.

Programming Challenges

1. Expand SequenceRoutine.pm to include the routines you listed in exercise.

2. Use CGI.pm to create and process an input form for a hypothetical Smith-Waterman search program. The search program is invoked from the Unix system by the following command:

   ```
   sw [-g <gap_penalty>][-m <matrix_name>] [-r] <file_name>
   ```

   (r is a simple flag to invoke repeat masking) and it returns a plain text file for the results.

3. Use text fields and whatever other HTML widgets you might need to create the input form. Return the output as unformatted plain text.

Part III

Advanced Perl

Chapter 9

References

In Chapter 5, we saw that we could not pass more than one array to a subroutine, because Perl flattens the arrays into a single list. The answer was to use a special construct called a reference. Perl references are similar to the concept of pointers in other languages. A reference is simply a scalar that refers to another variable, be that variable a scalar, an array, or a hash. References not only make it possible to pass multiple arrays (and hashes) to a subroutine, but it makes possible complex data structures like arrays of arrays.

9.1   Creating References

The mechanism for creating a reference to any variable is simple. References are created by using a backslash in front of the variable prefix.

```
$scalarRef = \$scalar;
$arrayRef =  \@array;
$hashRef =   \%hash;
```

The scalar variable now holds a reference to the original variable, which is now called the referent.

To get the value of the referent, we have to dereference the variable that contains the reference. We do that by prefixing another $ to the reference.

```
$scalar = 1;
$sRef = \$scalar;        #reference to a scalar
print $$sRef;            #prints 1
```

Perl Programming for Biologists,   D. Curtis Jamison
ISBN 0-471-43059-5   Copyright © 2003 Wiley-Liss, Inc.

The double dollar sign tells the Perl interpreter to dereference the value stored in $sRef back into a scalar value. Dereferencing an array reference is similar, but we have to make sure that we are specifically asking for an array:

```
@array = ("a", "b", "c");
$aRef = \@array;        #reference to an array
print @$aRef            #prints abc
```

We use a similar syntax to dereference a hash back from a hash reference:

```
$hRef = \%hash;         #reference to a hash
print %$hRef;           #prints the hash
```

Once a reference has been dereferenced, we can treat it just like the standard type. For example, we can assign the contents of an array reference to another array:

```
@newArray = @$aRef;
```

However, if we have a reference to an array, we don't have to copy it back into another array to get at a specific value in the referenced array. That would be wasteful. Instead, Perl allows us to access information inside the dereferenced array just like any other array by replacing the @ with a $ and adding an index. However, the precedence rules force us to add some grouping brackets around the hash reference:

```
print $$aRef[0];        #wrong: prints
print ${$aRef}[0];      #right: prints a
```

Because the dereferencing syntax can get confusing, Perl gives us a shortcut called the arrow operator. The arrow operator is a minus sign followed by a greater-than sign (which looks like an arrow), and it takes a reference on the left side and an array index on the right. This tells Perl to dereference the reference and fetch the value indicated by the index:

```
print $aRef=>[0];           #right: prints a
```

It is helpful to think of the arrow operator as meaning "what the reference points to."

Values inside a hash reference can also be accessed using the arrow operator. In this case, we put the hash index on the right:

```
print $href=>{"key"};
```

9.2   ref()

Because references all are scalars, it is often useful to be able to ask what type the referent was. We can do this using the ref command

```
ref($reference)
```

The ref function returns a string telling us what the type of referent the reference refers to. The string is the name of the type in all capital letters like "SCALAR," "ARRAY," or "HASH." If we pass ref() a scalar by mistake, then the string value is undefined. The ref function is also called when we try to print a reference. Thus, the code

```
print $aRef . "\n";
```

prints out

```
ARRAY(0xd8e0)
```

which is simply the return value from the ref function with the memory location of the referent appended.

Because a reference is simply a scalar, we can pass the reference to a subroutine and the copy of the reference will still point at the referent:

```
@myArray = ('a', 'b', 'c');
$arrayRef = \@myArray;
print $arrayRef . "\n";
&mySub($arrayRef);

sub mySub {
    $newRef = shift;
    print "subroutine" . $newRef . "\n";
}
```

When we execute this code, we get the following output:

```
perl refer.pl
ARRAY(0xd95c)
subroutine ARRAY(0xd95c)
```

The fact that the appended memory location is the same tells us we are dealing with the same array in both the subroutine and the main program. If we had a copy, the two numbers would be different. Thus we can be sure that any changes we make to the array in the subroutine will show up in the main program.

9.3   Anonymous Referents

Perl allows us to create a reference to an array or a hash directly, without going through the step of actually creating the array or hash first. Arrays (and hashes) created this way are called anonymous arrays and are useful for passing reference to subroutines.

We can create an anonymous array reference by using a list-style initialization, replacing the parentheses with square brackets, and assigning directly into the reference scalar:

```
$aRef = [1, 2, 3];
```

which has exactly the same effect as

```
@array = (1, 2, 3);
$aRef = \@array;
```

but takes fewer lines (and some people think it looks better also). The square brackets tell Perl that we want an anonymous array, and so it returns a reference rather than a list. Similarly, we can create an anonymous hash by enclosing the hash list in curly braces rather than parentheses:

```
$hRef = {gold=>1, silver=>2, bronze=>3};
```

is equivalent to writing

```
%hash = (gold=>1, silver=>2, bronze=>3);
$hRef = \%hash;
```

No matter how the hash reference is created, we can access the content by using the arrow operator:

```
print "The gold goes to number $hRef=>{gold}";
```

will find the value associated with the "gold" key in our anonymous hash.

As we will see in the next chapter, anonymous hashes are especially useful for writing object-oriented Perl.

9.4 Tables

Another major use for an anonymous reference is to create multidimensional tables. For example, let's revisit the sequence list we used to create a hash table in Chapter 3. There we were first saving a list of gene names in an array. But, typically, we want to store many data items describing the same gene. For example, we might have the gene name, a GenBank ID, information about where the GenBank record came from, and a size for the coding region. We want to use this data to create a table that looks like Figure 9.1.

We can create the table using an array of arrays. First, we will create an array for each of the five rows. Each of the row arrays will contain the four names we want to store:

Gene Name	GenBank ID	Source	Size (bp)
CAPZA2	XM_004969	predicted	2337
TFEC	NM_012252	mRNA	1805
CFTR	M28668	mRNA	6129
LOC51691	NM_016200	mRNA	537
LOC56311	XM_004978	predicted	1063

Figure 9.1 A table of gene data

```
@array1 = ('CAPZA2','XM_004969','predicted','2337');
@array2 = ('TFEC','NM_012252','mRNA','1805');
@array3 = ('CFTR','M28668','mRNA','6129');
@array4 = ('LOC51691','NM_016200','mRNA','537');
@array5 = ('LOC56311','XM_004978','predicted','1063');
```

Next, we create another array to hold references to each of the five arrays:

```
@aliases = (\@array1, \@array2, \@array3, \@array4, \@array5);
```

Now the @aliases array contains references to the arrays that hold all the data. Pictorially, we might think of the table looking like Figure 9.2.

With that picture in mind, it is relatively easy to see how we can get at the data stored in the table. If we look at a specific entry in the @aliases array, say the item at index 2, we get back the reference to the array we stored there which for index 2 is the array that contains the information for the CTRF gene. We can then follow the reference and look at a specific index (like index 1) in the second array to find the alias stored there:

```
$row = $aliases[2];
$GBID = $row->[1];
```

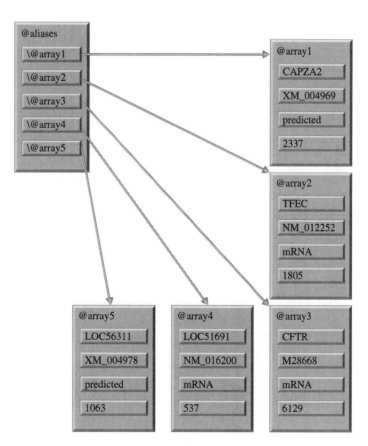

Figure 9.2 An array of array references

or, in one fell swoop:

```
$GBID = $aliases[2]=>[1];
```

or, even more simply

```
$GBID = $aliases[2][1];
```

and, because tables like this are so common, Perl will assume the arrow operator when it comes across a pair of array indices together.

The creation of a specific named array to represent each row might get a little tedious, especially if we want to include an entry for all 2771 genes on chromosome 7. It is even more onerous if we realize that we aren't ever going to use those array variables again. But we can simplify our lives (and our code) greatly by making use of anonymous arrays when we build our table:

```
@aliases = (['CAPZA2','XM_004969','predicted','2337'],
            ['TFEC','NM_012252','mRNA','1805'],
            ['CFTR','M28668','mRNA','6129'],
            ['LOC51691','NM_016200','mRNA','537'],
            ['LOC56311','XM_004978','predicted','1063']);
```

Chapter Summary

- A reference is Perl's version of a pointer.

- References are created using the \ in front of a valid variable name.

- The ref() command tells use what type of variable the referent is.

- Anonymous array references can be created using the square brackets [ ] instead of parentheses to enclose the list.

- Anonymous references to hashes can be created using the curly braces { } instead of parentheses.

Exercises

1. Why are anonymous referents important?

2. Explain the relationship between a reference and a referent.

3. Which of the following expression properly dereferences the third value in the array reference?

   a. $aref[2]

   b. $$aref[2]

   c. ${$aref}[2]

   d. ${$aref[2]}

e. $aref->(2)

f. $aref->[2]

g. $aref->{2}

Programming Challenge

1. Create a table using the microarray data parser created in Programming Challenge 6.1.

Chapter 10

Object-Oriented Programming

10.1 Introduction to Objects

There are two major paradigms for writing computer code. Thus far, the example code presented has followed the procedural programming paradigm. Our variables have been defined at the beginning, our code has been arranged in functions and subroutines, and the program flow has been more or less linear. In many regards, the code we have seen looks much like a recipe or a laboratory protocol. In essence, our code has been organized into a single file with a structure that looks like Figure 10.1.

The second programming paradigm is object-oriented programming (OOP). In OOP, the variables and code are encapsulated into logical groupings called classes. The organization of an OOP design looks more like Figure 10.2. Note that the code is split across multiple files. Each file represents a class, and all the code within a class has a common purpose.

- variable declarations
- main program
- functions and subroutines

Figure 10.1 Procedural code layout

Perl Programming for Biologists, D. Curtis Jamison
ISBN 0-471-43059-5 Copyright © 2003 Wiley-Liss, Inc.

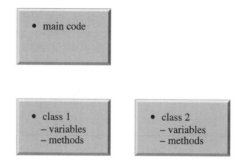

Figure 10.2   Object-oriented code layout

Both the procedural and object-oriented design approaches to writing programs are valid, and the approach to choose depends upon preference. Procedural code is typically used for short programs because the design phase is much simpler and shorter when compared with the complex design considerations for creating object-oriented programs. However, the simplicity of the procedural approach is lost when programs reach too large of a size, and for these larger programs OOP has a definite advantage of being easier to maintain and modify. In the end, the amount of code to write is roughly the same, the only difference is the organization of the program.

10.1.1   The OOP Approach

The OOP approach attempts to model a system as a set of interacting objects. The objects group and organize the behaviors of the complex systems. If we view object-oriented design as an organizational issue, the design principles become language independent: we can write object-oriented code in any language, just like we can write procedural code in any language. We just have to have the right state of mind.

The first step in getting into the right state of mind is to understand what constitutes an object. An object is comprised of attributes and actions. Attributes are the things that describe the object (which we store in variables). Actions are the tasks the object can do (which are encapsulated in chunks of code called methods). Together, the attributes and actions create a unique object.

The object-oriented approach to programming is an attempt to duplicate the way things interact in the real-world. For example, we can use OOP to model a real world object like a flower by writing a flower class that contains all the important information and features associated with being a flower. We would create variables to hold attributes like color, flower shape, numbers of petals, and so forth. We would also write methods that contained code to interact with those variables to model processes that change our flower object in specific ways, like wilting. Best of all, if we write the class code correctly, we can use our class to represent multiple types of flowers, because all flowers have a color, and all flowers wilt.

When we write object-oriented code, we try to reflect the structure of an object in the code. Attributes and actions are grouped together into structures known as classes. Class variables contain the attributes, and class methods contain the actions. The code in a class is a description of the form an object should take.

It is important not to confuse classes and objects. The class is the general description, and the object is the actual occurrence, or instance, of the class. A single class can describe many different objects. For example, we might write a class that describes the attributes and actions associated with a fruit. Later, we can create instances of the fruit class with different attributes and we will have objects representing an apple, an orange, and a pear. Similarly, dogs, cats, and cows are instances of the animal class, and the vehicle class can be instanced with car, boat, and train objects.

10.1.2 Class Design

When we design a class, there are three steps we need to follow. In order, we need to

1. decide what types of objects make up the system to be modeled;

2. determine which objects belong together; and

3. describe the common components of each group of objects.

When we finish this process, each description constitutes a class. For example, we can go to the botany department and make a list of all the types of plants we see there. These might include such things as:

- sunflowers

- orange trees

- oak trees

- roses

- wheat

- corn

Examining the list, we see that there are some items that we can group together:

- sunflowers, roses

- orange trees, apple trees

- wheat, grass

We then describe the common elements within these groups, and we end up with three classes: the flower class, the tree class, and the grass class. Note that the grouping we have here is not the only possible grouping, nor even a scientifically correct one (roses may be closer to trees than sunflowers on a cladogram), but instead represents how we want to model the data.

When we describe a class, we look for attributes and actions that are common to all members of the class. Thus, for the flower class, we can create variables for color, number of petals, number of leaves, and so forth. With enough variables, we can fully describe both a rose and a sunflower within the same class.

For methods, we look for active processes that alter those variables. For example, all flowers eventually wilt. The wilting process involves losing petals and leaves, and changing the color of the flowers. All these actions can be encapsulated into methods: dropPetals(), dropLeaves(), changeColor(). The whole wilt process can then be written as an aggregation of other methods:

```
wilt() {
  dropPetals(random());
  dropLeaves(random());
  changeColor("black");
}
```

Building methods by aggregation is an example of code reuse, and is the chief advantage of the OOP methodology. The complexity of the larger methods are reduced, and the smaller methods can be reused by many methods. The short, simple methods are easier to understand and maintain.

10.1.3   Inheritance

Another mechanism of code reuse is inheritance. Quite often, two distinct classes might share some common characteristics. For example, our Flower class would probably share many similarities to the Tree or Grass class. We can save time and energy by abstracting the generalities into a base class (say the Plant class), and then building upon that foundation using inheritance to create subclasses.

In many ways, the relationship between superclasses and subclasses is similar to the relationship in taxonomy. As you move from the kingdom (Plantea) down through genus and species (*Toxicodendron radicans*), you are adding characteristics that distinguish members of that taxonomic level from others, while retaining the characteristics of the higher level. Anthophytes and gymnosperms still share the common characteristics of all spermatophytes, even though they have characteristics that differentiate the two groups. Similarly, the methods and attributes of the superclass are inherited by all the derived subclasses, even though they might have different features that separate them as distinct classes.

10.2   Perl Objects

Even though Perl is not typically considered an object-oriented language, it is still possible to write object-oriented Perl code. There are some rudimentary object-oriented functions, but mainly we adhere to a set of rules and conventions that allow us to write object-oriented code. These rules and conventions can be broken, but to do so simply creates a piece of code that is less useful and harder to maintain.

There are three rules to writing object-oriented Perl, as defined by Larry Wall (the creator of Perl). In order to write or use Perl objects we need to remember that

1. classes are packages,

2. methods are subroutines, and

3. objects are blessed referents.

10.2.1   Rule Number One

This rule simply says that when we are creating our object-oriented Perl code, we keep all the information for a particular class inside a package. As we saw in Chapter 8, packages group similar subroutines together for inclusion in a larger program, and they also serve to create distinct namespaces within a program. Many aspects of packages are quite similar to classes, so we can equate a package with a class. The package name becomes the name of the class.

For example, suppose we want to take the SequenceRoutines.pm module we created in Chapter 8 and rewrite it into object-oriented Perl. The first step would be to create a file and create a package. The package name will be the class name, and the class name should define the type of objects the class defines. Therefore, we will call our class "`Sequence`" because that is what the class will contain

```
package Sequence;
```

Equating a class with a package also implies that each class is in a separate module, and therefore in a separate file. Again, this corresponds well with the paradigm of object-oriented programming, making it easier to maintain our code. Thus we should call our file "`Sequence.pm.`"

10.2.2   Rule Number Two

Rule two is also straightforward. It means that the code we write for methods is simply arranged into subroutines, and we call the subroutine when we want to invoke a method. Because the subroutines are grouped together in packages, if we equate a package with a class, by extension we equate the package subroutines with the class methods. In practice, this approach approximates the object-oriented approach quite well. Remember that a package creates a namespace, and a subroutine within that package is distinct from any subroutines in other packages, even if they appear to have the same name.

We already know two methods we want to use, RandomSeq and ReverseComplement. So we create subroutines with those names.

```
sub RandomSeq {
  ## code for RandomSeq
}

sub ReverseComplement {
  ## code for ReverseComplement
}
```

There are some minor changes that we will have to make to the actual code of the methods, because of some of the implications of rule three. Thus, we will leave the body of the methods empty for the moment.

10.2.3   Rule Number Three

Blessing a referent is the actual trick to creating object-oriented Perl code. The referent is some sort of data structure (usually a hash) that contains data of a specific sort. The bless command marks the referent as belonging to a particular class or package. After the referent has been blessed, we can use it's reference to access any of it's data *and* any of the methods of the class it has been blessed into.

The structure of the bless command is quite simple. It takes two arguments, a reference and a string containing the package name

```
bless($reference, "package_name")
```

The command attaches an invisible flag to the data structure referred to by the reference. That flag contains the string for the package name, and indicates that the data structure belongs to the specified package, and has all the rights and privileges of a member.

So, to create an object of our Sequence class, we would simply create a reference to a data structure that contains our sequence information, and invoke bless() on it:

```
$seqRef = \%seq;
bless $seqRef, "Sequence";
```

Now, not only can we use $seqRef as a reference to get to the data stored in the %seq hash, we can also use it to invoke the methods we declared as part of the "Sequence" package:

```
$seqRef=>RandomSeq();
$seqRef=>ReverseComplement();
```

Once we have blessed a referent into a class, Perl understands that the arrow operator followed by a subroutine refers to a class method.

Thus far we've avoided stating exactly what sort of data structure we're going to bless. In the Sequence example, we've used an associative array, but bless()

will accept any reference, and so our referent can be any data structure: arrays, type-globs, even scalars. However, a hash reference is by far the most common structure used.

The biggest advantage to using an associative array is the built-in data identifiers. Remember when we access a hash reference, we use the key to get to the value:

```
$seqRef=>{name}
```

which returns whatever value is associated with the "name" key. Thus, a data structure using a hash has a built-in data identifier, as long as we are careful to make the names meaningful.

Since we are going to use a hash, we need to decide what data items we are going to keep track of for our sequence objects. This is an important decision, because we want to be sure to track everything the methods in our class might need access to, since an object is supposed to be self-contained. To keep things simple, we'll only track three attributes: the GenBank ID, the name, and the sequence. So now we can expand our code to include setting the data

```
%seq = (_id=> "", _name=> "CTRF", _seq=> "ATTGG...");
$seqRef = \%seq;
bless $seqRef, "Sequence";
```

Note that we have used an underscore in front of each key. This is purely a stylistic convention. The underscore serves to remind us that the keys are internal to the blessed data structure.

Recall that in Chapter 9 we explored methods of making our code more efficient using references to anonymous arrays. The same issues apply to making objects: we don't want to have to create a named array for every object we're going to bless into the Sequence class. Again, we can simplify our object code by using anonymous hashes

```
$seqRef = {_id=> "", _name=> "CTRF", _seq=> "ATTGG..."};
bless $seqRef, "Sequence";
```

Now that we have our data structure defined, we can go back and look at our methods and define exactly how they should work and what they should do. The definitions become the interface to our class, and control how a user of our class will interact with it. Any reasonable (or even unreasonable) set of definitions is allowed, as long as we make sure the rules are available for our users to understand.

10.2.4 Methods

Back in Chapter 8 we created a package of subroutines for sequence analysis. One of those routines created a random sequence (perhaps to use to test a new search comparison algorithm). The original RandomSeq subroutine returned a random sequence that was then stored in a variable. In the object-oriented world, it is reasonable to expect that the user wants the current sequence object to contain a random sequence. So our method will replace the current object attributes with a random sequence. We will still look for a length and default to 40 if it is unspecified.

To turn our procedural subroutine into a class method, we rewrite our code so it looks something like this:

```
sub RandomSeq {
    @nucleotides = ('a', 'c', 'g', 't');
    my $self = shift;
    my $length = shift || 40;
    $self=>{_id} = "0000";
    $self=>{_name} = "Random Sequence";
    $self=>{seq} = "";
    for (my $i = 0; $i < $length; $i++) {
        my $base = $nucleotides[int(rand(4))];
        $self=>{_seq} .= $base;
    }
}
```

Compare the object-oriented code shown here with the procedural code from Chapter 8. The very first change we note is that there is a mysterious extra parameter that wasn't specified in our user interface that is getting shifted off the argument list. The name of the variable we are shifting it into, and the way that we are using it later in the code, give us clues to what this variable is. It appears to be a reference to the current Sequence object. But where did it come from?

Actually, Perl put it there for us. Whenever we use an object to invoke a class method, Perl prepends a reference to the current object into the argument list. That way, our class methods know what object called them. After the shift operation, $self becomes another reference to the hash we blessed in $seqRef, and we can manipulate the data in the hash. Thus, when we adjust the value pointed to by $self->{_id} we are really adjusting the value in $seqRef->{_id}.

In fact, the lines altering _id and _name are the next difference between the SequenceRoutines subroutine and the Sequence method. Although the two attributes are not specifically the sequence, we still want to alter them to reflect the change we are going to make in the sequence. An object needs to be treated rather holistically, and the id and name are as much of a part of the object as the actual sequence.

Finally, we alter the sequence itself. We write the new sequence directly into the data structure using the seq key, and we no longer worry about returning a value. The object value is changes when we finish writing into $self->{seq}.

The ReverseComplement subroutine changes similarly. However, in this case, we decide that we would rather return a new object containing the reverse complement of the sequence stored in the current object. We can write the new method as follows:

```
sub ReverseComplement {
    $self = shift;
```

```
    my %rev;
    $rev{_id} = "000";
    $rev{_name} = $self->{_name} . "reverse complement";
    $rev{_seq} = reverse($self->{_seq});
    $rev{_seq} ~= tr/actg/tgac/g;
    return bless \%rev, ref($self);
}
```

Again, the first thing in our argument list is a reference to the current object. We use that reference to gain access to the attributes of the current object. We create a new associative array to hold the details of the reverse complemented sequence object. Finally, we return a reference to a blessed Sequence object. Note that we used the ref command, giving it $self as an argument. The ref() command returns the type of the referent, and when given an object reference it returns the name of the class the object belongs to. In this case, the string would be "Sequence" because that is the name of the class.

Now our users can write

```
bless $seqRef, "Sequence";
$revSeqRef = $seqRef->ReverseComplement();
```

and create a new sequence object and its complement.

10.2.5 Constructors

An issue with using bless() is that it will happily bless any data structure into any class. Thus, someone with evil intentions could actually write a piece of code that looked like

```
$carRef = {_make=> "Pontiac",  _model=> "Firebird",
_engine=> "V8"};
bless $carRef, "Sequence";
```

Obviously this would create a problem when we go to invoke the ReverseComplement method. Even if there is a defined object that is the reverse complement of a Firebird (a Yugo perhaps), the method would fail because the code in the Sequence::ReverseComplement() method is going to be looking for the _seq attribute that the car data structure doesn't have. And, while an evil user would deserve what they got, we also have to worry about our users who might make an honest mistake by forgetting to initialize a variable or by accidentally blessing a DNA object into a RNA class.

One way to avoid confusion and make life easier for people using your class is to provide a constructor. A constructor is a method that instantiates an object by creating the data structure, blessing the data structure into the class, and returning a reference to the new object. By convention, this method is called new().

We would write the new() method for the Sequence class simply by encapsulating the object creation code we've already seen into a new() method.

The user will then create a Sequence by invoking the new() method with the appropriate arguments:

```
$seqRef = Sequence::new("Sequence", "", "CTRF", "ATTGG...");
```

and then use it as a normal Sequence object. The code for the new method will look something like this:

```
sub new {
   my ($class, $id, $name, $seq) = @_;
   my $ref = {_id=>$id, _name=>$name, _seq=>$seq};
   return bless $ref, $class;
}
```

The code is very straightforward. We simply put the arguments into the right place in our hash, and then we bless the hash into a Sequence object. Note that the string "Sequence" is the first argument to our constructor, and we use that string as the class name argument to the bless command. This is another one of the Perl object-oriented programming conventions. We don't have to do it this way, but it makes our constructor work better, especially when the constructor is called using the arrow notation

```
$seqRef = Sequence->new("", "CTRF", "ATTGG...");
```

Notice the difference between the module-like invocation of the new method using the double colons and the more object-oriented version with arrow operator. In the latter instance, the arrow automatically places the name of the package as the first argument, similar to when it prepended the reference to the current object in the argument list to a normal class method. Using the arrow operator and building constructors makes using the class a little easier.

A class can have multiple constructors. By strict definition, any method that returns a newly blessed object is a constructor, so in fact our ReverseComplement method is actually a constructor. Similarly, we might decide it makes more sense to have RandomSeq be a constructor as well:

```
sub newRandomSequence {
   my $class = shift;
   my $length = shift || 40;
   my %self;
   $self->{_id} = "0000";
   $self->{_name} = "Random Sequence";
   $self->{seq} = "";
   for (my $i = 0; $i < $length; $i++) {
      my $base = $nucleotides[int(rand(4))];
      $self->{_seq} .= $base;
   }
   return bless \%self, $class;
}
```

So now rather than creating a new Sequence object and overwriting it with a random sequence, we can create it directly:

```
$rSeq = Sequence->newRandomSequence(70);
```

10.2.6   Accessors

Earlier, we noted that when we create a hash to store attributes, it is customary to put an underscore in front of the hash key to remind us that they are internal to the blessed data structure. Although we can write code that uses those internal variables directly, it is usually better to provide methods that set or return the value of the attribute. This way we can preserve the internal integrity of the object data structure, and we can also hide the internal workings of our class.

Methods that access the data in an object are not surprisingly called data accessors. By convention, a class supplies an accessor for every attribute that can be set by the user of that class. Accessors can be used to fetch the value of the attribute, set a new value, or both. Usually, the accessor is named so that it is clear what attribute is being manipulated.

Our sequence class has three attributes, so we want to create accessors that will return the value of each of the accessors. The accessor for the id attribute might look something like:

```
sub ID {
  my $self = shift;
  return $self=>{_id};
}
```

The accessor is simplicity itself. We shift the reference to the object off the argument list, and then use the argument to access the value stored in the hash keyed by the string _id. Now to print the ID of the sequence, we would simply write

```
print $seqObj=>ID;
```

The accessors for the other attributes would be similar.

10.2.7   OOP Versus Procedural

As a final note, let's pull together the complete Sequence.pm class file and compare it with the SequenceRoutines.pm module from Chapter 8:

```
package Sequence;

my @nucleotides = ('a', 'c', 'g', 't');

sub new {
  $ref = {_id=>$_[1], name=>$_[2], seq=>$_[3]};
  return bless $ref, $_[0];
}

sub newRandomSequence {
  my $class = shift;
  my $length = shift || 40;
```

```
    my %self
    $self=>{_id} = "0000";
    $self=>{_name} = "Random Sequence";
    $self=>{seq} = "";
    for (my $i = 0; $i < $length; $i++) {
        my $base = $nucleotides[int(rand(4))];
        $self=>{_seq} .= $base;
    }
    return bless \%self, $class;
}

sub ReverseComplement {
    my $self = shift;
    my %rev;
    $rev{_id} = "000";
    $rev{_name} = $self=>{_name} . "reverse complement";
    $rev{_seq} = reverse($self=>{_seq});
    $rev{_seq} ~= tr/actg/tgac/g;
    return bless \%rev, ref($self);
}

sub ID {
    my $self = shift;
    return $self=>{_id};
}

sub Name {
    my $self = shift;
    return $self=>{_name};
}

sub Sequence {
    my $self = shift;
    return $self=>{_seq};
}

1;
```

The amount of code in the two files is about the same, although Sequence.pm has a little more due to the constructor, the accessors, and the extra lines needed to maintain the entire object. However, the real savings comes in the main code, where our use of object-oriented programming makes our code much easier to understand. For example, imagine a simple program that creates a random sequence, complements it, and then prints out a Fasta library containing both sequences.

Using Sequence.pm our code looks like

```
use Sequence;

$forward=>newRandomSequence(80);
$reverse = $forward=>ReverseComplement();

print ">" . $forward=>ID . $forward=>Name . "\n";
```

```
print $forward=>Sequence . "\n";
print ">" . $reverse=>ID . $reverse=>Name . "\n";
print $reverse=>Sequence . "\n";
```

whereas the same program using SequenceRoutine.pm would look like

```
use SequenceRoutine;

$forwardSeq = RandomSeq(80);
$forwardID = "000";
$forwardName = "Random Sequence";
$reverseSeq = ReverseComplement($forwardSeq);
$reverseID = "000";
$reverseName = "RandomSeq reverse complement";

print ">" . $forwardID . $forwardName . "\n";
print $forwardSeq . "\n";
print ">" . $ReverseID . $reverseName . "\n";
print $reverseSeq . "\n";
```

Both programs perform the same task and produce the exact same output. But the object-oriented version uses less code, and is cleaner when handling the data (using two variables rather than six). The object-oriented code would be even cleaner if we applied more advanced object-oriented techniques like data access methods and keyed constructors.

In the long run, using object-orientated program techniques over procedural programming techniques is largely a matter of preference. Typically, object-oriented techniques are adopted when creating large programs that are going to be used for long periods of time, whereas the procedural is quicker and easier for which to write short, quick programs. Object-oriented programming also gives us the huge advantage of being able to use class libraries like Bioperl, which we will see in the next chapter.

Chapter Summary

- Object-oriented programming attempts to model a system as a set of inter-acting objects.

- A class is a general description (or code).

- An object is a specific instance of a class.

- Attributes are the data that describes an object.

- Actions are the methods an object can perform.

- Subclasses inherit from superclasses, and extend the capabilities of the class.

- Perl classes are packages.

- Perl methods are subroutines.

- Perl objects are blessed referents.

For More Information

Conway, D. (1999) *Object Oriented Perl*. Manning, Greenwich, UK.

```
perldoc perlobj
```

Exercises

1. Explain when it is better to write object-oriented code rather than procedural.

2. Explain the difference between a class and an object.

3. Design a sequence class. Include in the description the attributes and methods needed.

4. Why do we create a new() function for all our classes?

5. What is the arrow operator?

6. Of the following list, what would be a class and what would be an object? Justify your answers.

   a. tiger

   b. tree

   c. ponderosa pine

   d. gene

   e. CTRF

Programming Challenges

1. Implement the sequence class from Exercise 3, above.

2. Write a Perl class that keeps track of the full taxonomy and the common names of animal species.

Chapter 11

Bioperl

Every bioinformaticist who has been in the business for any length of time has a directory on their computer containing Perl scripts representing tools for various computational tasks. If you were to catalog the programs, you would find many that fall into a specific subset of tasks, and that the same task has been solved in a myriad of different ways. It has been said that every bioinformaticist has written a program to reverse complement Fasta files at least once, and most of us have written it two or three times.

Fortunately for the bioinformaticist, there is Bioperl. Bioperl is a collection of modules that facilitates the development of bioinformatics applications. The software is maintained by a dedicated group of bioinformatic programmers who generously donate their time and energy. The latest information about the project can be found at the www.Bioperl.org Web site.

Bioperl is strongly object oriented. Each module represents a class complete with constructors, data accessors, and methods. Including the Bioperl modules gives access to many bioinformatic classes, including classes for modeling sequences and alignments, communicating with databases, and with other programs. Figure 11.1 lists the major components of Bioperl.

11.1 Sequences

The main classes that most of Bioperl revolves around are the sequence manipulation classes. There are several sequence classes that are available for use, depending upon the desired goals of you program. For example, the Large-Seq class is specialized for maintaining genomic-sized (>100 Mb sequences)

Perl Programming for Biologists, D. Curtis Jamison
ISBN 0-471-43059-5 Copyright © 2003 Wiley-Liss, Inc.

Category	Distribution or Module	Comment
Sequences	Bio/Seq.pm	main sequence storage class
	Bio/Seq/	specialized sequence storage classes
	Bio/SeqFeature/	sequence features classes
	Bio/SeqIO/	sequence file format converters
	Bio/LiveSeq/	sequence that changes over time
	Bio/Annotation.pm	sequence database links and literature references
	Bio/Variation/	sequence polymorphisms
Alignments	Bio/SimpleAlign.pm	sequence alignment tool
	Bio/AlignIO/	aligned sequence file format converters
Database connectivity	Bio/DB/	remote database communication protocols
	Bio/Index/	local database access tools
Tools	Bio/Tools	bioinformatic algorithms

Figure 11.1 Select Bioperl modules and distributions

whereas the LiveSeq class is geared toward storing sequences that have features that change over time. However, the default, general purpose sequence representation is Seq.

A Seq object is very straightforward to create. We simply call the new method, supplying several keys value pairs representing the sequence data:

```
$seq = Bio::Seq->new(-seq => 'ATCGT',
                     -desc => 'Sample sequence',
                     -display_id => 'something',
                     -accession_number => 'GB_ID',
                     -moltype => 'dna');
```

First, note that all the keys start with a – , which indicates they are parameter names for arguments to the Bio::Seq module (this is patterned after the Unix command line options convention). The key names are pretty much self-explanatory about what type of information the value encodes. The only one that is even mildly tricky is the moltype, which can be 'dna', 'rna', or 'protein'. All values are supplied as string values.

Once a Seq object is created, we have many possible methods we might perform with it. For example,

```
## print as a fasta file
print '> ' . $seq->accession_number() . ' ' .
      $seq=>desc() . "\n";
for ($i = 0; $i" < length; $i+=70) {
  print $seq=>subseq($i, $i+70) . "\n";
}
```

which we can print out a Fasta file with little muss and fuss. The first print statement creates the Fasta defline, using the accession_number() method and the desc() methods to get the database accession number and the molecule description. Note that we don't have to remember that the description is stored in a hash keyed by the string `"-desc"` because the desc() method remembers that for us: this type of method is known as a data accessor method because it accesses the data for us.

Next we have a for loop that iterates over the sequence, printing out 70 bases per line. The 70 bases are extracted from the sequence using the subseq() method. The method is similar to the substr() command in that it extracts a subsequence from the main sequence, but the supplied variables are the start and endpoint.

We can also automatically convert sequences:

```
$protSeq = $seq=>translate();
```

translates a nucleic sequence object into a protein sequence object. The behavior of the translate() method can be controlled by a variety of variables, including specifying the frame and codon translation tables.

11.2 SeqFeature

If we consider a sequence, we note that there are always subsequences of greater importance than other subsequences. For example, an ALU repeat or a promoter region might be more interesting to us than the entire sequence. Most of the large biology databases have recognized this, and for most entries the databases provide some form of annotation.

For example, in the GenBank record for the working draft sequence NT_007930 we find the following section:

```
FEATURES                Location/Qualifiers
     source             1..5669875
                        /organism="Homo sapiens"
                        /db_xref="taxon:9606"
                        /chromosome="7"
     STS                33..234
                        /standard_name="D7S3100"
                        /db_xref="UniSTS:186668"
     gene               151..5576
                        /gene="MUC3B"
                        /db_xref="LocusID:57876"
                        /db_xref="MIM:605633"
```

(plus a lot more entries). This is the feature table, and it tells us exactly what biologically relevant features exist in the sequence record, along with their positions. For example, we see there is an STS found within the sequence: D7S3100 can be found between bases 33 and 234 of this sequence entry.

Obviously, it would be worthwhile to be able to navigate through these entries. The SeqFeature module provides just such a mechanism. When we get a Seq object from a database, we also get a list of the features stored in a list within that Seq object. We can access those features via the Seq::top_SeqFeatures() or the Seq::all_seqfeatures() methods, both of which return a list of SeqFeature references. We can then iterate through the list, examining the features for one aspect or another:

```
my @features = $mySeq=>all_seqfeatures();
foreach $feature (@features) {
  //do something with the features
}
```

All features have a start and a stop position, defined relative to the parent sequence. The start and stop are retrieved from the SeqFeature using the start() and end() methods respectively. So, if we pretend that $feature contains the feature description for the D7S3100 STS defined above, $feature=>start() would return 33, and $feature=>end() would return 234.

The feature table works on the idea of tags. A tag is closely related to a key, in that a feature is made up of tag-value pairs that describe the feature. The primary tag is the keyword used by GenBank to describe the overall feature: STS, gene, etc. The secondary tags begin with a / and are separated from the associated value by an equal sign. Going back to our D7S3100 example, the primary tag would be "STS", while there are two secondary tags called "standard_name" and "db_xref."

We access the tags through a couple of methods. The primary_tag() method returns the primary tag, while the all_tags() returns a list containing the secondary tags. We can use that list to get the values associated with the tag using the each_tag_value() method:

```
foreach $tag ( $feat->all_tags() ) {
  print "Feature has tag ", $tag, "with values, ",
  join(' ',$feat->each_tag_value($tag)), "\n";
}
```

Note that the each_tag_value() method also returns a list, because a tag can have more than one value (as seen by the multiple db_xref tags in the gene feature).

11.3 Annotation

One special type of sequence feature is an annotation. Annotations are brief descriptions that convey some biological information about the sequence. For example, we might want to link our sequence to some experimental data we found during a literature search. The Bio::Annotation provides exactly such a facility.

An annotation object can contain four types of data: a brief description, comments, links to other objects, and references to literature. The description is a standard text string. Comments, DBLinks, and References are classes with the Bio::Annotation hierarchy.

We use the new method to create an annotation:

```
my $ann = Bio::Annotation=>new('-description'='text');
```

The new method only accepts the description. Comments, DBLinks, and References need to be added using the add_Comment(), add_DBLink(), and add_Reference() methods, respectively. The description text should be a single, brief line of text. Use the Comment attribute to add longer comments:

```
$ann=>add_Comment(Bio::Annotation::Comment=>
    new('-text' =>'comment1'));
```

We use the Comment::new() method with a string to create a long comment (perhaps about the experimental method used or the abstract of the new paper). We can add as many Comments as we like to the Annotation.

Similarly, we use the DBLink::new() method to create a new external database link (using "-database" and "-primary_id" to initialize the name of the database and the UID, respectively) and the Reference::new() method to create a literature reference (using "-authors", "-title", "-location", and "-start" to initialize the author list, the article title, the journal, and the page number, respectively).

For example. we could create a new annotation like this:

```
my $DBLink = Bio::Annotation::DBLink=>new(
        -database => "PubMed",
        -primary_id => "11099254");
my $lRef = Bio::Annotation::Reference=>new(
        -authors => "Jamison DC, Thomas JW, Green ED.",
        -title => "ComboScreen facilitates the multiplex
hybridization-based screening of high-density clone
arrays.",
        -location => "Bioinformatics 2000 Aug;16(8)",
        -start => 678);
my $comment = Bio::Annotation::Comment=>new(
        -text => "abstract in PubMed");
my $ann = BioAnnotation=>new(
        -description => "ComboScreen paper");
```

11.4 Sequence I/O

While the Bio::Seq class is powerful, just using the class by itself may not be the best answer for most programs. We probably don't want to hard-code our sequences into our scripts, creating new features and annotations by hand. Instead, we will probably want to read the Seq objects in from database files that we have downloaded from a database. Bioperl provides us with a set of SeqIO objects that save us from having to create code to ingest and parse databases into our programs. SeqIO classes exist for all the major database formats, including GenBank, EMBL, Fasta, and PIR.

The SeqIO object also takes care of writing data in a specific format. For example, to reformat a file containing EMBL records into a file of Fasta records, we could write

```
$in = Bio::SeqIO=>new(-file => "inputfile",
                -format => 'EMBL');
```

```
$out = Bio::SeqIO=>new(-file => ">outputfile",
                       -format => 'Fasta');
while (my $seq = $in=>next_seq()) {
  $out=>write_seq($seq);
}
```

The first two lines set up the input and output filters. The filenames are strings with the same conventions as arguments to the open command, which in fact they are. The format argument contains a string specifying the format the SeqIO object will read or write. The next_seq() command is used to iterate over the EMBL sequence records in the input file, whereas the write_seq() command outputs each EMBL record as a Fasta record.

The object returned by the next_seq() command is a Seq object. Thus, we can use the Seq object read from the file just like any other Seq object.

As useful as SeqIO is, more often than not we are interested in getting only a single sequence from a database. The Bio::DB modules save us from having to manually download sequences. These modules will communicate with remote databases like GenBank or SwissProt to fetch sequence records across the Internet and turn them into Seq objects that we can use in our programs:

```
use Bio::Seq;
use Bio::DB::GenBank;

$gb = new Bio::DB::GenBank();
while (shift @ARGV) {
  $seqs{$_} = $gb=>get_Seq_by_id($_);
}
```

This code creates a hash (%seqs), which contains a bunch of Seq objects, keyed by id (which we conveniently read in from the command line using the @ARGV array). The get_Seq_by_id() method takes care of establishing a communications channel to GenBank, requesting a specific record, and then converting the record into a Seq object. We can improve upon our code by using the batch fetch mode:

```
use Bio::Seq;
use Bio::DB::GenBank;

$gb = new Bio::DB::GenBank();
$seqio = $gb=>get_Stream_by_batch(@ARGV);
while ($seq = $seqio=>next_seq()) {
  $seqs{$seq=>display_id} = $seq;
}
```

This code does the exact same thing (creates a hash of Bio::Seq objects keyed by id), except the sequences are gotten all at once rather than one at a time. We still create the DB::GenBank object, but instead of individual Seq objects we fetch a SeqIO object using the get_Stream_by_batch() method. We then iterate through the SeqIO object using the next_seq() method. This code is tremendously more efficient than the previous example, because we only open a channel to GenBank once.

11.5 Cool Tools

Bioperl contains many algorithms that can be invoked within your program. These utilities are contained in the Tools distribution. For example, the Tools::SeqStats class computes many useful descriptive statistics about sequences, including the molecular weight and residue occurrence counts. Similarly, Tools::RestrictionEnzyme will find all the restriction sites in a sequence.

Using the Tools modules simply requires instancing a new Tools object with a Seq object as the argument:

```
use Bio::Seq;
use Bio::DB::GenBank;
use Bio::Tools:OddCodes

$gb = new Bio::DB::GenBank();
$seqio = $gb=>get_Stream_by_batch(@ARGV);
while ($seq = $seqio=>next_seq()) {
  $code = Bio::Tools::OddCodes=>new($seq);
  print $seq=>id . "\n";
  print $seq=>seq . "\n";
  print $code=>charge() . "\n\n";
}
```

The OddCodes class computes things like hydropathy and charge for a protein sequence. After we fetch a batch of Seq objects, we iterate over them creating a new OddCodes object. Then we print out the sequence id, the sequence, and the charge for each residue. The first entry in out output would look something like:

```
sequenceid
ACDEFGH
NNAANNC
```

In addition to utilities, the Tools distribution includes modules for parsing output from search tools like BLAST and HMMER. The parsers are generally used when creating automated annotation pipelines. For example, to parse through the results of a BLAST search we would write:

```
use Bio::Seq;
use Bio::Tools::BPlite;

$resFile = shift;
$rep = Bio::Tools::BPlite(-fh => $resFile);
$rep=>query;
while (my $hit = $rep=>nextSbjct()) {
  $hit=>name;
  while (my $hsp = $hit=>nextHSP()) {
    $hsp=>score();
  }
}
```

The BLAST results file is passed to the script through the @ARGV array, and a new BLAST parser is created using the name of the result file. The query() method digests the report and creates a list of BLAST hits, which we then iterate over. The next_Sbjct() method gives a BLAST hit object that contains a list of BLAST HSP objects, which we can again iterate over, retrieving the score for all HSPs.

11.6 Example Bioperl Programs

To conclude our exploration of Bioperl, the following program is presented as an example of using Perl and Bioperl in a real laboratory environment. The program was written to support the required informatics for a sequencing lab. The desire was to quickly generate primer pair candidates for use in STS mapping.

11.6.1 Primer.pl

This program was written to support the required informatics for a sequencing lab. The desire was to quickly generate primer pair candidates for use in STS mapping. We use Bioperl modules to fetch the sequences from GenBank.

```perl
#! /usr/bin/perl
#
# primers.pl
#
# Reads a list of accession numbers from the command line,
# fetches the sequences from GenBank, and then generates a
# set of primers somewhere in the first 500 bases. We show a
# preference for coding regions if we can manage it.
#
# 13Nov1998
# DCJ

# import required modules
use strict;
use Bio::Seq;
use Bio::DB::GenBank;
use Primer3;

# set up variables
my %sequences;
my $key;
my $feature;

# Fetch sequences from GenBank, keyed by accession
my $gbConnect = new Bio::DB::GenBank();
my $seqIO = $gbConnect->get_Stream_by_acc(@ARGV);
while (my $tempSeq = $seqIO->next_seq()) {
  $sequences{$tempSeq->display_id} = $tempSeq;
```

```
   }

   # iterate over sequences
   foreach $key (keys(%sequences)) {

      # set arbitrary start point
      my $start = 50;
      my @features = $sequences{$key}=>top_SeqFeatures();

      # try to start in CDS if we can
      foreach $feature (@features) {
       if ($feature=>primary_tag eq 'CDS') {
          if ($feature=>start() < 400) {
            $start = $feature=>start();
          }
          last;
        }
      }

      #search for primers
      my $primer = Primer3=>new($key,
         $sequences{$key}=>subseq($start, $start + 500));
      print "$key\nLeft\t\t\tRight\t\t\tLength\tPenalty\n";
      while ($primer=>getNextPair()) {
         if (($primer=>penalty() < 9) && ($primer=>productGC() <
   60)) {
            print $primer=>leftOligo()."\t" .
   $primer=>rightOligo() . "\t" .
            $primer=>productLength(). "\t" .
    $primer=>penalty(). "\n";
         }
      }
      print "\n";
   }
```

After the comment block that explains what the program is used for, and any assumptions we've made, the first few lines of code import the modules we are going to use. The strict module makes sure our code is written to a good standard, and the Bio::Seq and Bio::DB::GenBank provide storage for the sequences and connection to GenBank, respectively. Finally, we use a special module called Primer3, which provides a connection and interface to the Primer3 software. We will examine this module closely in the next section.

The next few lines of the program declare some variables. Because we are using strict, we need to make sure that all our variables are scoped to the local namespace. If we weren't using strict, we could simply have let these variables autovivify as globals.

Next we use the Bio::DB::GenBank module to fetch the sequences. First we set up a new connection to GenBank, then we send the entire argument list to the GenBank server to fetch the sequences in batch mode. The sequences are brought back in a Bio::SeqIO object, which we iterate over using the next_seq() method.

For each sequence, we first figure out the leftmost position allowable for the primer. The arbitrary start point is 50, just to make sure we are well inside the sequence. We get the feature table from the sequence object, and iterate over the features looking for the first CDS. If we find it with 400 bp of the sequence start, we use that, otherwise we stick with the arbitrary 50 bp start.

Finally, we do the primer search and print out the results. Here we create a new Primer3 object by giving the constructor a 500 bp subsequence. We will see how in the next chapter, but for now accept that the Primer3 constructor runs the primer3 program and returns an object containing several primer pairs, which we can iterate over using the getNextPair() method. We iterate over the primer pairs, printing out our report:

```
% primers.pl AC013798
AC013798
Left                      Right                    Length   Penalty
CCTCCTGGACAACCTGTGTT  TGAAGTCAGGGGACATAGGG      280      0.0823
CCTCCTGGACAACCTGTGTT  AGGCCAGTAGACTGGGTGTG      298      0.1758
CCTCCTGGACAACCTGTGTT  GGTGTGAAGTCAGGGGACAT      284      0.1852
TTCCCGCATCTCTTAGCAGT  AGGCCAGTAGACTGGGTGTG      209      0.1962
CTTCCCGCATCTCTTAGCAG  GACACTAGTGGCAAGGAGGC      226      0.2362
```

Most of the primers.pl program is extremely simple. The real guts and power of the program lie in the classes and the methods we call. The next section examines the Primer3 module, which is similar to many Bioperl modules.

11.6.2   Primer3.pm

The Primer3 module is a Perl class that interfaces with the Primer3 program (a C program that runs under Unix). Although not a Bioperl module, it contains similar design parameters and would be very simple to turn into a Bioperl module.

```
#
# Primers.pm
#
# Simplified class for primer3.
#
# Retrieves and manages primer3 output. Note: many primer3
# options not implemented (using defaults) and others are
# hard-coded. This is not a generic primer3 interface!!!
#
# 13Nov1998
# DCJ

package Primer3;

# import a few modules
use FileHandle;
use IPC::Open3;
```

```perl
# non-standard defaults: For any options not in
# this list, we use the generic primer3 default
# values.
my $primer3_prog = '/usr/local/bin/primer3';
my %definitions = (PRIMER_PRODUCT_SIZE_RANGE =>"200-450");

## Constructor
sub new {
# setup variables
  my ($class, $name, $seq) = @_;
  my %results;

  # create BoulderIO command stream
  my $command ="PRIMER_SEQUENCE_ID =$name\nSEQUENCE =$seq\n";
  my $arg;
  foreach $arg (keys(%definitions)) {
    $command .= "$arg=$definitions{$arg}\n";
  }
  $command .= "=\n";

  # send command to primer3 program
  my ($read, $write) = (FileHandle=>new, FileHandle=>new);
  my $pid = open3($write, $read, $read, "$primer3_prog");
  print $write $command;
  $write=>close;

  # read results from primer3 into hash
  while ($_ = $read=>getline) {
    chomp;
    my ($key, $value) = split("=");
    $results{$key} = $value;
  }
  return bless(\%results, $class);
}

## Iterator: Set index to next primer pair
sub getNextPair {
  my $self = shift;
  if (exists $self=>{_CURRENT}) {
   # already counting
    $self=>{_CURRENT}++;
    if ($self=>{_CURRENT} <= $self=>count()) {
      # valid primer pair
      return 1;
    } else {
      # we've run out of primer pairs
      return 0;
    }
  } else {
    # initialize counter
    if ($self=>count()) {
      # we have primers to iterate over
      $self=>{_CURRENT} = 0;
      return 1;
```

```
      } else {
        # we have no primers to work on
        return 0;
      }
    }
}


# Note for accessors: The first primer pair is officially
# primer pair 0. Each attribute in the hash is named with
# the primer pair number appended (or embedded) in the name
# *EXCEPT* for primer pair 0. Thus PRIMER_PAIR_PENALTY is
# the penalty for the first pair, PRIMER_PAIR_PENALTY_1 is
# the the second, and so forth. This leads to the odd little
# if statement to append the underscore and number to every
# primer pair key except the first one.

## Accessor: Number of primer pairs
sub count {
  my $self = shift;
  return int(keys(%{$self})/20 - 1);
}

## Method: Calculate GC content of product
sub productGC {
  my $self = shift;

  # find the start position of the current left primer
  my ($leftKey) = "PRIMER_LEFT";
  if ($self=>{_CURRENT}) {
    $leftKey .= "_$self=>{_CURRENT}";
  }

  # create substring for product
  my ($start) = split(',', $self=>{$leftKey});
  my $length = $self=>productLength();
  my $prodSeq = substr($self=>{SEQUENCE}, $start, $length);

  # calculate GC percentage rounded to two decimal places
  my $GC = $prodSeq =~ tr/GC/GC/;
  return int(($GC/$length)*10000)/100;
}

## Accessor: Penalty
sub penalty {
  my $self = shift;
  # create hash key for current pair
  my $key = "PRIMER_PAIR_PENALTY";
  if ($self=>{_CURRENT}) {
    $key .= "_$self=>{_CURRENT}";
  }
  return $self=>{$key};
}

## Accessor: product length
```

```
     sub productLength {
       my $self = shift;

       # create hash key for current primer pair
       my $key = "PRIMER_PRODUCT_SIZE";
       if ($self=>{_CURRENT}) {
         $key .= "_$self=>{_CURRENT}";
       }
       return $self=>{$key};
     }

     ## Accessor: left oligo
     sub leftOligo {
       my $self = shift;

       # create hash key for current primer pair
       my $key = "PRIMER_LEFT";
       if ($self=>{_CURRENT}) {
         $key .= "_$self=>{_CURRENT}";
       }
       $key .= "_SEQUENCE";
       return $self=>{$key};
     }

     # Accessor: right oligo
     sub rightOligo {
       my $self = shift;

       # create hash key for current primer pair
       my $key = "PRIMER_RIGHT";
       if ($self=>{_CURRENT}) {
         $key .= "_$self=>{_CURRENT}";
       }
       $key .= "_SEQUENCE";
       return $self=>{$key};
     }
     1;
```

The first step in creating a new module is to declare the name of the module using the package command. We then import a couple modules, FileHandle and IPC::Open3. Finally, to finish the setup, we define a pair of package variables: the $primer3_prog is the fully qualified program name (meaning it has the full Unix path), and %definitions is a hash that contains values for the primer3 parameters that we wish to use. Aside from redefining the product size, our program will use the default values associated with primer3.

The rest of the Primer3.pm file consists of subroutines that make up the methods of the class. The first subroutine is new(), which serves as a constructor for the Primer3 object.

The constructor is relatively simplistic, taking only two arguments: the sequence name and the sequence string. The first thing the constructor does is to shift those arguments (along with the Perl-supplied class name) into local variables. We also define a hash to hold our program results.

Next, we create the command we will supply to the Primer3 program. The command has a unique structure based upon the BoulderIO format, which consists of a keyword followed by an equal sign and the value associated with the keyword. We represent the command as a string containing the keywords and values, appending the arguments from the %definitions hash (which we have cleverly designed to hold the parameter values indexed by the actual parameter keyword).

The next section is the only part of our module that isn't immediately recognizable, because we have used an uncommon extension to the Perl language. The open3 command is from the IPC::Open3 module, and it allows us to safely open a program pipe for both reading and writing, something the standard open command won't do. The exact use of open3 is detailed in the perlipc section of the perldocs; suffice it here to say that the open3 creates reading and writing filehandles to the command supplied. We can then print our command to the filehandle referenced by $write and read the results from the filehandle referenced by $read. The results are also returned in BoulderIO format, so we simply have to split the incoming lines on the equal sign to get key-value pairs for our results hash. Blessing a reference to the hash into our class gives us the return value for our constructor.

The getNextPair() method is a special type of method called an iterator. An iterator assumes that you have a list of values and want to step through them sequentially. However, rather than returning a value, the iterator keeps track of which primer pair we are currently working with, and returns a true value if it can advance to a new primer pair. So if we were working on the second primer pair, after we make a call to getNextPair() we would be working with the third primer pair.

The way we keep track of which primer pair we are working on is simple. We keep a value in our hash (keyed by the index string "_CURRENT") that contains an integer. The integer corresponds to the current primer pair, and to advance to the next primer pair we increment current. There are two special cases to watch for: when we are done iterating, and when we haven't started iterating yet. The first situation is easy, we simply check our incremented _CURRENT value against the count of primers, returning a 0 if we've incremented past the last one. The second situation is also easy to look for because, before we begin iterating, the _CURRENT key-value doesn't exist. The only tricky part is that in the Primer3 output the primer pairs are numbered from 0, so we set the _CURRENT value to 0. Now all our accessors can use the value associated with _CURRENT to find the right value to return.

At the beginning of the accessor methods, there is a rather lengthy comment about the nature of the Primer3 output. This comment helps orient future maintainers of the module, alerting them to look for some special code. In general, it is always a good idea to document the structure of any files you are reading, just in case the structure of the file changes and breaks your code.

The first accessor is a method we saw used in the getNextPair() method. The count method returns the number of primer pairs returned from the Primer3 program. To get the count, we count the number of keys and divide by 20, because there are 20 lines of output per primer pair. There are also a few lines extra, so we turn the result into an integer, and then we subtract one to make the counter start from zero. This somewhat arcane formula was determined empirically by examining the output of the primer3 program.

The next method calculates the CG content of the product defined by the current primer pair. First, we build a key to get the value associated with the PRIMER_LEFT tag, appended an underscore and the primer number if needed, as detailed in the comment that started the accessor section. Then we extract the position information from the string. We also get the length of the product through another accessor. Then we create a temporary string by extracting the substring that represents the product from the string that represents the sequence. Finally, we count the number of Gs and Cs using the tr operator, and perform a calculation that returns the percentage CG rounded to two decimal places.

The remaining accessors (Penalty, productLength, leftOligo, and rightOligo) all follow the same pattern. First, the proper key is constructed, appending or embedding the proper index number from the _CURRENT value, and then returning the value associated with the key.

Chapter Summary

- Bioperl contains much of the code needed for bioinformatics programming.

For More Information

```
www.Bioperl.org
perldoc perlipc
```

Exercises

1. From the Bioperl documentation, explain the difference between the various sequence classes.

2. Which Bioperl modules might you use in a program to

   a. perform a SNP search

   b. create a phylogenetic tree

   c. translate genomic sequences from GenBank into a Fasta library

3. What other applications might you use Primer3.pm for?

Programming Challenges

1. Write a script for any of the programs listed in Exercise 2.

2. Write a script using Bioperl that will accept any number of accession numbers to be fetched from GenBank and output the residue-by-residue hydropathy for each. Some considerations:

    *   some sequences might be nucleic;

    *   the hydropathy string should be intercalated with the sequence string, not exceeding 70 characters per line;

    *   hint: you've seen 95% of the script in the examples.

3. Turn Primer3.pm into a real Bioperl module. Make allowances for the need to change the parameters, and create all the required accessors.

Appendix A
Partial Perl
Reference

This is a partial listing of Perl functions and keywords used in this book. For a complete listing, see Wall or perldoc perlfunc.

Chapter 3

Functions for arrays

pop	Removes and returns the last value in an array
push	Puts a new value at the end of the array
shift	Removes and returns the first value in an array
unshift	Puts a new value at the front of the array

Functions for list data

join	Turns a list into a string
reverse	Reverses the order of a list
sort	Rearranges a list into a new order

Functions for hashes

delete	Completely deletes a key-value pair
exists	Return true if a key exists
keys	Returns the keys in a list
values	Returns the values in a list

Perl Programming for Biologists, D. Curtis Jamison
ISBN 0-471-43059-5   Copyright © 2003 Wiley-Liss, Inc.

Chapter 4

Keywords related to control flow

last	Stop executing the loop immediately
next	Go to the next iteration of the loop immediately
redo	Do the same iteration of the loop over again

Chapter 5

Keywords related to scoping

my	Restrict a variable to the local scope

Keywords related to subroutines

return	Return a value from a subroutine
sub	Define a subroutine
wantarray	Check whether a subroutine is being used in a scalar or an array context

Chapter 6

Functions for strings

chomp	Removes the record-separator character (usually "\n") from the end of a string
index	Returns the location of the first occurrence of a substring within a larger string
length	Returns the length of a string
m//	Regular expression match operator
reverse	Reverses a string
rindex	Same as index, but start from the right
s///	Regular expression substitution operator
split	Breaks a string into a list at the specified characters
substr	Returns a specified substring from with a larger string
tr///	Translation operator
y///	Translation operator

Chapter 7

Input and output functions

die	Prints a string and exits the program
print	Prints a string

Functions for filehandles, files, or directories

close	Disconnects a file handle from a file or process
open	Connects a file or process to a file handle

Chapter 8

Keywords related to Perl modules

package	Create a name for a module
use	Read a module into the program

Chapter 9

Keywords related to classes

bless	Make an array into an object of a particular class
ref	Returns the type of a reference

Appendix B
Bioinformatics File Formats

The world of bioinformatics is extreme in the number of competing and non-interchangeable formats, all invented to represent the same or highly similar data. Definitions for data interchange conventions like CORBA and XML are therefore frightfully large, because they attempt to take into account all the various nuances and templates covered by the competing data formats.

This appendix presents several of the more popular and stable data formats, with samples suitable to be used in writing parsers for data munging. However, this is a snapshot, current of the writing, and may not accurately reflect the current state of the format. For that reason, wherever possible, a primary source has been cited.

GenBank

The GenBank format is a standardized informational format. It was developed by the National Center for Biotechnology Information, the National Library of Medicine, and the National Institutes of Health, and is the standard display format for the GenBank databases. The format consists of a set of nested keyword identifiers and free-text entries. GenBank records are delimited by a pair of forward slashes // on a single line.

The GenBank format is designed to be human readable and convey both bibliographic and feature information about a sequence. While the format is parsable, the information is also available in the ASN.1 format.

Perl Programming for Biologists,   D. Curtis Jamison
ISBN 0-471-43059-5   Copyright © 2003 Wiley-Liss, Inc.

```
LOCUS       CFA315401    4934 bp    mRNA           MAM      02-AUG-2001
DEFINITION  Canis familiaris mRNA for multidrug resistance protein 2 (mrp2
            gene), transcript variant 1.
ACCESSION   AJ315401
VERSION     AJ315401.1  GI:15130909
KEYWORDS    alternative splicing; mrp2 gene; multidrug resistance protein 2.
SOURCE      dog.
  ORGANISM  Canis familiaris
            Eukaryota; Metazoa; Chordata; Craniata; Vertebrata; Euteleostomi;
            Mammalia; Eutheria; Carnivora; Fissipedia; Canidae; Canis.
REFERENCE   1  (bases 1 to 4934)
  AUTHORS   Conrad,S., Viertelhaus,A., Orzechowski,A., Hoogstraate,J.,
            Gjellan,K., Schrenk,D. and Kauffmann,H.M.
  TITLE     Sequencing and tissue distribution of the canine MRP2 gene compared
            with MRP1 and MDR1
  JOURNAL   Toxicology. 156 (2-3), 81-91 (2001)
  MEDLINE   21108656
REFERENCE   2  (bases 1 to 4934)
  AUTHORS   Conrad,S., Racky,J., Orzechowski,A., Hoogstraate,J., Gjellan,K.,
            Kauffmann,H.M. and Schrenk,D.
  TITLE     Transcript variants of the canine MRP2 gene
  JOURNAL   Unpublished
REFERENCE   3  (bases 1 to 4934)
  AUTHORS   Kauffmann,H.M.
  TITLE     Direct Submission
  JOURNAL   Submitted (23-JUL-2001) Kauffmann H.M., Food Chemistry
            /Environmental Toxicology, University of Kaiserslautern,
            Erwin-Schroedinger-Strasse 56, D-67663 Kaiserslautern, GERMANY
COMMENT     related sequence Y18220.
FEATURES             Location/Qualifiers
     source          1..4934
                     /organism="Canis familiaris"
                     /db_xref="taxon:9615"
                     /tissue_type="Liver"
     gene            3..4637
                     /gene="mrp2"
     CDS             3..4637
                     /gene="mrp2"
                     /function="drug conjugate transporter"
                     /note="alternative splicing"
                     /codon_start=1
                     /evidence=experimental
                     /product="multidrug resistance protein 2"
                     /protein_id="CAC48162.1"
                     /db_xref="GI:15130910"
                     /translation="MLEKFCNSTFWNSSFLDSPEADLPLCFEQTVLVWIPLGFLWLLA
                     PWQLLHVYRTKIKRSSITKLYLAKQVLVGFLLILAAIELVLVLTEDSGEATVPAIRYT
                     NPSLYLGTWLLVLLIQYSRRWCVQKDSWFLSLFWILSILCGSFQFQTLIRTLLKDSNS
                     NLAYSCLFFIGYALQILVLILSAFSEKDASSNNPSFTASFLSSITFSWYDSIVMKGYK
                     QPLTLEDVWDVDEQITTKALVSKFEKYMVEELQKARKTLQKQQQRNTQGKSGERLHDL
                     NKNQSQSQDILVLEEVKKKKKKSGTTEKFPKSWLVKSLFKTFYVILLKSFLLKLVFDL
                     LTFLNPQLLKLLISFANDPDMYVWTGYFYSVLFFVVALIQSLCLQSYFQMCFMLGVNV
                     RTTIMASIYKKALTLSNQARKQYTIGETVNLMSVDAQKLMDVTNFIHLLWSNVLQIAL
                     SIYFLWAELGPSILAGVGVMILLIPVNGLLASKSRAIQVKNMKNKDKRLKIMNEILSG
                     IKILKYFAWEPSFKNQVHELRKKELKNLLTFGQMQSVMVFLLYLTPVLVSVITFSVYT
                     LVDSNNVLDAEKAFTSITLFNILRFPLSMLPMVISSLLQASVSRERLEKYLGGDDLDT
                     SAIRRDSSSDKAVQFSEASFTWDRDSEATIRDVNLEIMPGLMVAVVGTVGSGKSSLMS
                     AMLGEMEDVHGHITIKGTIAYVPQQSWIQNGTIKDNILFGSELDEKRYQQVLEACALL
                     PDLEVLPGGDLAEIGEKGINLSGGQKQRISLARATYQNSDIYVLDDPLSAVDAHVGRH
                     IFNKVLGPNGLLKGKTRLLVTHSIHFLPQVDEIVVLGNGTILEKGSYNTLLAKKGLFA
                     KILKAFTKQTGPEGEATVNEDSEEDDDCGLMPSVEEIPEEVASLTMKRENSLHRTLSR
                     SSRSRSRHQKSLRNSLKTRNVNTLKEEEEPVKGQKLIKKEFIQTGKVKFSIYLKYLRA
                     IGWYLIFLIIFAYVINSVAYIGSNLWLSAWTNDSKAFNGTNYPASQRDMRIGVYGVLG
                     LAQGVFVLMANLLSAHGSTHASNILHRQLLNNILQAPMSFFDTTPTGRIVNRFAGDIS
                     TVDDTLPQSLRSWILCFLGIVSTLVMICTATPVFIIVIIPLSIIYVSIQIFYVATSRQ
```

```
                    LKRLDSVTRSPIYSHFSETVSGLSVIRAFEHQQRFLKHNEVGIDTNQKCVFSWIVSNR
                    WLAVRLELIGNLIVFFSSLMMVIYKATLSGDTVGFVLSNALNITQTLNWLVRMTSEIE
                    TNIVAVERINEYIKVENEAPWVTDKRPPPGWPSKGEIRFNNYQVRYRPELDLVLRGIT
                    CDIRSMEKIGVVGRTGAGKSSLTNGLFRILEAAGGQIIIDGVDIASIGLHDLREKLTI
                    IPQDPILFSGSLRMNLDPFNHYSDGEIWKALELAHLKTFVAGLQLGLSHEVAEAGDNL
                    SIGQRQLLCLARALLRKSKILIMDEATAAVDLETDHLIQMTIQREFSHCTTITIAHRL
                    HTIMDSDKIIVLDNGKIVEYGSPQELLRNSGPFYLMAKEAGIENVNSTSF"
BASE COUNT      1320 a    1135 c    1150 g    1329 t
ORIGIN
         1 tcatgctgga gaagttctgc aactctacgt tttggaactc ttcattcttg gatagcccag
        61 aagcggacct gccactttgt tttgagcaaa ctgttctggt gtggattccc ttgggtttcc
       121 tttggctcct ggccccttgg cagcttcttc atgtgtatag gaccaagatc aagagatctt
       181 ctataaccaa actctacctt gctaagcagg tgcttgttgg gtttcttctt attctagcag
       241 ccatagagct ggtccttgta ctcacagaag actctggaga agccacagtc cccgccatta
       301 gatacaccaa tccaagcctt tacctgggca catggctcct ggttttgctg atccaataca
       361 gcaggcgatg gtgtgtacag aaggattctt ggttcctgtc tctattctgg attctctcaa
       421 tactctgtgg tagtttccaa tttcagactc tgatccggac actcttaaag gacagcaatt
       481 ctaacttggc ttactcctgc ctgttcttca tcggctatgc actacagatc ctggtcctga
       541 tcctatcagc attttcagaa aaagatgcct cctcaaataa tccatcattc acggcctcat
       601 ttctgagtag cattacgttt agttggtatg acagcattgt tatgaaaggc tacaagcaac
       661 ctctgacact ggaagatgtg tgggatgttg atgaacagat tacaaccaag gcactggtca
       721 gcaagtttga aaaatatatg gtagaagagc tgcagaaggc cagaaagacc ctccagaaac
       781 agcaacagag gaacacccag gggaagtctg gagaaaggct gcatgacttg aacaagaatc
       841 agagtcaaag ccaagatatc cttgttctgg aagaagttaa aaagaaaaaa aagaagtctg
       901 ggaccacaga aaagtttccc aagtcctggt tggtcaagag tctcttcaaa actttctatg
       961 tcatactctt gaaatcattc ctactgaagc tggtgtttga ccttctcacg ttcctgaatc
      1021 ctcagctgct gaagttgctg atctcctttg caaatgaccc agacatgtat gtgtggactg
      1081 ggtatttcta ttcggtcctc ttctttgttg tggctctcat ccagtctctc tgccttcaga
      1141 gctactttca aatgtgcttc atgttgggtg taaacgtacg gacaaccatc atggcttcca
      1201 tatacaagaa ggcgctgacc ctttccaacc aggccaggaa gcagtacacc attggagaaa
      1261 cagtgaacct gatgtctgtg gatgctcaga agctcatgga tgtgaccaac ttcattcatc
      1321 tgctgtggtc aaatgttctc cagattgctt tatctatcta cttcctgtgg gcagagctgg
      1381 gaccctccat cttagcagtt gttggggtga tgatactcct aattccagtt aatgggctac
      1441 ttgcctctaa gagtagagct attcaggtaa aaaatatgaa gaataaagac aaacgtttaa
      1501 agatcatgaa tgaaattctc agtgggatca agatcctgaa atattttgcc tgggaacctt
      1561 cattcaaaaa ccaagtccac gaacttcgga agaaagagct caagaacctg ctgaccttcg
      1621 ggcagatgca gtctgtaatg gtgtttctct tatacttaac tccggtcttg gtgtctgtga
      1681 tcacgttttc agtttacact ctggtggaca gcaataatgt tttggatgca gagaaggcat
      1741 tcacctccat caccctcttc aatatcctgc gctttcccct aagcatgctc cccatggtaa
      1801 tctcctcact gctccaggcc agcgtttcca gagaacgcct ggaaaagtac ttgggagggg
      1861 atgacttaga cacatccgcc attcgacgtg acagcagttc tgacaaagct gtgcagttct
      1921 cagaggcctc cttcacctgg gaccgggact cggaagccac aatccgagat gtgaacctgg
      1981 agattatgcc aggccttatg gtggctgtgg tgggcactgt aggctctggg aagtcttcct
      2041 tgatgtcagc catgctggga gaaatggaag atgtccatgg gcacatcacc atcaagggca
      2101 ccatagccta cgtcccacag caatcctgga ttcagaatgg caccataaag gacaacatcc
      2161 tttttggatc cgagttggat gaaaagagat accagcaggt gctagaagcc tgtgccctcc
      2221 taccagactt ggaagtgctg ccgggaggag acctggctga gattggagag aagggtataa
      2281 atcttagtgg gggtcagaag cagcggatta gcctggccag agctacctat cagaattcag
      2341 acatctatgt tctggatgac cccctgtcag ctgtggatgc tcatgtggga agacatattt
      2401 tcaataaggt cttgggtccc aatggcctat tgaaaggcaa gactcgtctc ttggttacac
      2461 atagcattca ctttcttccc caagtggatg agattgtggt tctggggaat ggcaccatct
      2521 tggagaaggg atcctacaac actctgctgg ccaagaaagg attgtttgct aagattctga
      2581 aggcattcac aaaacagacg ggtcctgaag gagaggccac agtcaatgag gacagtgaag
      2641 aagatgatga ctgtgggctg atgcccagtg cctgaggaat ccctgaggaa gtggcctcct
      2701 tgaccatgaa aagagagaac agccttcatc gaacacttag tcgcagttcc aggtccagga
      2761 gcagacatca gaaatcccta agaaactctt tgaaaacccg gaatgtgaac actctgaagg
      2821 aggaggagga accagtgaaa ggacaaaaac taattaagaa ggaattcata caaactggaa
      2881 aggtgaagtt ctccatctac ctgaagtacc tacgagcaat aggatggtat ttgatattcc
      2941 tcatcatttt tgcctatgtg atcaattctg tggcttatat tggatccaac ctctggctca
      3001 gtgcttggac caatgactct aaagccttta atggcactaa ctatccagct tctcagaggg
      3061 acatgagaat tggcgtctat ggagttctgg gattagctca aggtgtgttt gtgctcatgg
      3121 caaatctctt gagtgcccat ggttccaccc atgcatcaaa catccttcac aggcaactgc
      3181 taaacaacat ccttcaagca cccatgagtt tttttgacac aacacccaca ggtcggattg
      3241 tgaacaggtt tgctggtgat atttccacag tggatgacac cctcccccaa tccttgcgca
      3301 gctggatatt gtgtttcctg ggaatagtca gcactcttgt catgatctgc acggccactc
      3361 cagtgttcat catcgtcatc attcctctta gcattattta tgtgtctatt cagatatttt
```

```
3421 atgtggctac ttcccgccag ctgaaacgtc tagactctgt caccagatcc ccaatttact
3481 ctcacttcag tgagacagtg tcaggtttgt ccgtcatccg tgcctttgag catcagcaga
3541 gatttctgaa acacaatgaa gtggggattg acaccaacca gaaatgtgtc ttttcctgga
3601 ttgtctccaa cagatggctt gcagttcgtc tggagctgat tgggaacttg attgtcttct
3661 tttcatccct gatgatggtt atttataaag ctaccctaag tggagacact gtgggctttg
3721 ttctgtccaa tgcacttaat atcacacaga ccctgaactg gctagtgagg atgacgtcag
3781 aaatagagac caacattgtg gctgttgaaa gaataaatga atacataaaa gtggaaaatg
3841 aggcaccctg ggtgactgat aagagacctc ccccaggttg gcccagcaaa ggggagattc
3901 ggtttaacaa ctaccaagtg cggtaccggc ctgaactgga tcttgtactg agagggatca
3961 cttgtgatat taggagcatg gagaagattg gtgtggtggg cagaacagga gctgggaagt
4021 catccttgac aaatggcctc ttcagaatcc tagaggctgc aggtggtcag atcatcattg
4081 atggggtaga tattgcttcc attgggctcc atgacctccg agaaaaattg accatcatcc
4141 cccaggatcc catcctgttc tctggaagcc tgaggatgaa tctagaccct tttaaccact
4201 actcagatgg ggagatttgg aaggccttgg agctggctca cctcaaaaca tttgtggctg
4261 gcctgcaact ggggttgtcc cacgaagtgg cagaggctgg tgacaacctt agcatagggc
4321 agaggcagct actgtgcctg gccagggctc tgcttcggaa atccaagatt ctgatcatgg
4381 atgaggccac tgctgcggtg gacctagaga ccgatcacct catccagatg accatccaaa
4441 gggagttctc ccactgcacg actatcacca ttgctcacag gctacacacc atcatggaca
4501 gtgacaagat aatagtccta gacaatggga agattgtaga gtatggcagc cctcaagaac
4561 tgctgagaaa ttcgggcccc ttttatttga tggccaaaga agctggcatt gaaaatgtga
4621 acagcacatc gttctgacag taggtcccat gggctgaaaa aggactataa gatcattcct
4681 tattttttg tgagagatac tacacagaag tttgtaaaat atacatttt gaagaaggat
4741 tgttatatcc agctacagcg gaccacccc aatcttgctt tgatgatccc acttcaattt
4801 tatctccttc atacttacct tcccagagat aactaacctg aattttgtga taatgatatc
4861 ctcctgcttt tcattttagt tttactactt ggtatgtacc cttaaacaag atatacctt
4921 tttaatttat gtga
//
```

ASN.1

The ASN.1 format for biological sequence information was also developed by the NCBI, and is closer to the native search and storage format. ASN.1 represents the data in a flexible hierarchical nested structure, which is straightforward to parse. Parsers for ASN.1 exist in many languages, including Perl and C. More information and a full description of the NCBI ASN.1 specification can be found at www.ncbi.nlm.nih.gov/Sitemap/Summary/asn1.html.

```
Seq-entry ::= set {
  level 1 ,
  class nuc-prot ,
  descr {
    comment "related sequence Y18220" ,
    update-date
      std {
        year 2001 ,
        month 8 ,
        day 2 } ,
    pub {
      pub {
        sub {
          authors {
            names
              std {
                {
                  name
                    name {
                      last "Kauffmann" ,
                      initials "H.M." } } } ,
            affil
```

```
                  str "Kauffmann H.M., Food Chemistry /Environmental Toxicology,
University of Kaiserslautern, Erwin-Schroedinger-Strasse 56, D-67663
Kaiserslautern, GERMANY" } ,
            medium other ,
            date
              std {
                year 2001 ,
                month 7 ,
                day 23 } } } } ,
     pub {
       pub {
         muid 21108656 ,
         article {
           title {
             name "Sequencing and tissue distribution of the canine MRP2 gene
compared with MRP1 and MDR1." } ,
           authors {
             names
               std {
                 {
                   name
                     name {
                       last "Conrad" ,
                       initials "S." } } ,
                 {
                   name
                     name {
                       last "Viertelhaus" ,
                       initials "A." } } ,
                 {
                   name
                     name {
                       last "Orzechowski" ,
                       initials "A." } } ,
                 {
                   name
                     name {
                       last "Hoogstraate" ,
                       initials "J." } } ,
                 {
                   name
                     name {
                       last "Gjellan" ,
                       initials "K." } } ,
                 {
                   name
                     name {
                       last "Schrenk" ,
                       initials "D." } } ,
                 {
                   name
                     name {
                       last "Kauffmann" ,
                       initials "H.M." } } } ,
             affil
               str "Food Chemistry/Environmental Toxicology, University of
Kaiserslautern, Erwin-Schroedinger-Strasse 52, D-67663 Kaiserslautern,
Germany." } ,
           from
             journal {
               title {
                 name "Toxicology." ,
                 iso-jta "Toxicology" ,
                 ml-jta "Toxicology" ,
                 issn "0300-483X" ,
                 jta "VWR" } ,
```

```
                imp {
                  date
                    std {
                      year 2001 ,
                      month 1 ,
                      day 2 } ,
                  volume "156" ,
                  issue "2-3" ,
                  pages "81-91" ,
                  language "eng" } } ,
            ids {
              pubmed 11164610 ,
              medline 21108656 } } } } ,
      pub {
        pub {
          gen {
            cit "Unpublished" ,
            authors {
              names
                std {
                  {
                    name
                      name {
                        last "Conrad" ,
                        initials "S." } } ,
                  {
                    name
                      name {
                        last "Racky" ,
                        initials "J." } } ,
                  {
                    name
                      name {
                        last "Orzechowski" ,
                        initials "A." } } ,
                  {
                    name
                      name {
                        last "Hoogstraate" ,
                        initials "J." } } ,
                  {
                    name
                      name {
                        last "Gjellan" ,
                        initials "K." } } ,
                  {
                    name
                      name {
                        last "Kauffmann" ,
                        initials "H.M." } } ,
                  {
                    name
                      name {
                        last "Schrenk" ,
                        initials "D." } } } } ,
            title "Transcript variants of the canine MRP2 gene" } } } ,
      source {
        org {
          taxname "Canis familiaris" ,
          common "dog" ,
          db {
            {
              db "taxon" ,
              tag
                id 9615 } } ,
          orgname {
```

```
          name
            binomial {
              genus "Canis" ,
              species "familiaris" } ,
          lineage "Eukaryota; Metazoa; Chordata; Craniata; Vertebrata;
Euteleostomi; Mammalia; Eutheria; Carnivora; Fissipedia; Canidae; Canis" ,
          gcode 1 ,
          mgcode 2 ,
          div "MAM" } } ,
      subtype {
        {
          subtype tissue-type ,
          name "Liver" } } } ,
    create-date
      std {
        year 2001 ,
        month 8 ,
        day 2 } } ,
  seq-set {
    seq {
      id {
        embl {
          name "CFA315401" ,
          accession "AJ315401" ,
          version 1 } ,
        gi 15130909 } ,
      descr {
        title "Canis familiaris mRNA for multidrug resistance protein 2 (mrp2
gene), transcript variant 1" ,
        molinfo {
          biomol mRNA } ,
        embl {
          div mam ,
          creation-date
            std {
              year 2001 ,
              month 8 ,
              day 2 } ,
          update-date
            std {
              year 2001 ,
              month 8 ,
              day 2 } ,
          keywords {
            "alternative splicing" ,
            "mrp2 gene" ,
            "multidrug resistance protein 2" } } } ,
      inst {
        repr raw ,
        mol rna ,
        length 4934 ,
        seq-data
          ncbi2na 'D39E882F790771BFE81DF4F7E8C95209A17947FBFE2407BDEBBA3D5FABF
5FE9D7A55FA49F7D3BB328508D088DF730501DC5F9C24AE7EFABF7DF3DC9253227AD7EC744821D
E882512D5653C8C450D425FC5EA44E9D7AFF9E350C49298EBBB120A3DFAF5EDDCF7A3DDD0C77BA
CBF50FD21DE35A11DF028490F707E9F1D797BDF4DA7391C48D7AD78D73493FD20023975D030D4D
3D1A5D3F78B24F1BF2FACE124FBCE029C424177847A08EEEA3BE38123C414291EB490BF800CCEB
2089E4829480857520124122811152A82DE880A79387E0420D22D02508CD7EF7A082F002000082D
EA144802FD50B5EBEB422DDF401FDCED31DF80D3D71E09EBBF85F746F5E0D749E782F9E375FE40
E15213B3BBA1EACFDCF6B5DF7FBEE9DD352DDDE5F489C7F40EE7D3BEAEC06C68414D3A7D4CC420
A67857F505294A092C453E8804B8178EDEE8E748274E8EE141F4F4DE7BAD03BDD48F9FCDCDC7D7
BA9227A857537C92BBEAB8E31D70F52F0EA71F97708B2273D2B000CE08302101BF0234E0E03DD2
EA34235E033FE5EA05F4F40050B5181F68202274205E785F6A48E4B7B0EBBF77CC7C1D6B7EBB7B
8D1BFD2FC477AE8490C3BFE8E488293D17534577D0CD799FD570939D54EB0DD7479D4A526FD488
197A00B1FA8AA387C844D653D86E124BDE1027B92F748A5D7D17A85A87682510D623B817A23CE5
297CEBA7BAEA47B29DEA0B7D7E3B494E7A880E823B53A91345342A45325C6D512435E8F483A453
```

0284135FFE8D62FA3802231492B9C825EE575C521FA0B9E5A8A217A788FA220AB3037CBAAB4824
9A3C97A5227173483D21373BDE8E155ED27BA39D3BA82133FD0C2B7EAD50E973E0290876DDFAF1
1324F47F7D542E8E23EEBDEA83A4537E882A35C411DE7A5080A3EFE708F78293D100486AD78288
A512D0E284B8208E387BA9E3952EE8A03578A0BA5D7E14E00888125F4D811F2D92F52B52892134
80D5C201DFE005683B811DE0A28A2814B80A1001C3C20A0F4C407A02B82F75371782C5C624328E
B3F8CF5D34FFE5CEE343DEE9F33E8D4177A74B9FA143877025FC3A47073525DD22A13883E9B73A
2F7A8F2742BBBFB9D3A40DDF8B953AF515393404D7D129079C04135F42454E2FFFE1104544ADA3
EE04AFE7AE33F512E8E115D550D7E649E8CFBBF5EA0CB491DFB4E3791A51D4BBD34DB4D3D77C93
CFCEEDCF48CFF3BA71F56527806DC877B4523550FC7747D2E212ED2BFB5B4D6E5FE24D2488FDE0
110E0BAA3E1141480EEDFF5E8FB75048E9F92F6DE89E3EA07E3EDF7FD3578E3AF3F302715C2E88
47BA9FEF7B50E47C3344485781E9CB8A386D203221413EE9EF808303831300BA00E2915EAE1E30
885D552BE95240AA23DAFC107142E6B169781E8DFB1E22A347EE33CA24E8823EBBAEA481289EA0
B4D7E103A5DF4835C8A792BAD234D3E3AAC8CF9F53EA75385D62003E14D3554A354D7BDDE825E2
8E0DC857FC1471D23AA23FA0A5FA27A745D004FEE9E97907AAFB5460BA48A7AE105F24CA922927
1EE5E94A9DE7DA03508F78D3A38A51E79AE85C8858D174D48E14D40A8BDD51E461CD14F9D129C4
4534E84B84230CB5C843A823EC8B3A495D081E7880F6A55FF3F8E940827A4F803B81244DBDE12C
AD53A9E00287308D3D7CFFFEE2231C4482FEC03313FF820A3EF33527126851550DF9FE38D51F43
FCDD7D31F17D52230705E0FFB8C38CD75E7FD3FCBFC71FACEC57C0423317FFC3F3B80'H } ,
            annot {
              {
                data
                  ftable {
                    {
                      data
                        gene {
                          locus "mrp2" } ,
                        location
                          int {
                            from 2 ,
                            to 4636 ,
                            id
                              gi 15130909 } } } } } ,
        seq {
          id {
            embl {
              accession "CAC48162" ,
              version 1 } ,
            gi 15130910 } ,
          descr {
            molinfo {
              biomol peptide } } ,
          inst {
            repr raw ,
            mol aa ,
            length 1544 ,
            seq-data
              ncbieaa "MLEKFCNSTFWNSSFLDSPEADLPLCFEQTVLVWIPLGFLWLLAPWQLLHVYRTKIKRS
SITKLYLAKQVLVGFLLILAAIELVLVLTEDSGEATVPAIRYTNPSLYLGTWLLVLLIQYSRRWCVQKDSWFLSLFWI
LSILCGSFQFQTLIRTLLKDSNSNLAYSCLFFIGYALQILVLILSAFSEKDASSNNPSFTASFLSSITFSWYDSIVMK
GYKQPLTLEDVWDVDEQITTKALVSKFEKYMVEELQKARKTLQKQQQRNTQGKSGERLHDLNKNQSQSQDILVLEEVK
KKKKKSGTTEKFPKSWLVKSLFKTFYVILLKSFLLKLVFDLLTFLNPQLLKLLISFANDPDMYVWTGYFYSVLFFVVA
LIQSLCLQSYFQMCFMLGVNVRTTIMASIYKKALTLSNQARKQYTIGETVNLMSVDAQKLMDVTNFIHLLWSNVLQIA
LSIYFLWAELGPSILAGVGVMILLIPVNGLLASKSRAIQVKNMKNKDKRLKIMNEILSGIKILKYFAWEPSFKNQVHE
LRKKELKNLLTFGQMQSVMVFLLYLTPVLVSVITFSVYTLVDSNNVLDAEKAFTSITLFNILRFPLSMLPMVISSLLQ
ASVSRERLEKYLGGDDLDTSAIRRDSSSDKAVQFSEASFTWDRDSEATIRDVNLEIMPGLMVAVVGTVGSGKSSLMSA
MLGEMEDVHGHITIKGTIAYVPQQSWIQNGTIKDNILFGSELDEKRYQQVLEACALLPDLEVLPGGDLAEIGEKGINL
SGGQKQRISLARATYQNSDIYVLDDPLSAVDAHVGRHIFNKVLGPNGLLKGKTRLLVTHSIHFLPQVDEIVVLGNGTI
LEKGSYNTLLAKKGLFAKILKAFTKQTGPEGEATVNEDSEEDDDCGLMPSVEEIPEEVASLTMKRENSLHRTLSRSSR
SRSRHQKSLRNSLKTRNVNTLKEEEEPVKGQKLIKKEFIQTGKVKFSIYLKYLRAIGWYLIFLIIFAYVINSVAYIGS
NLWLSAWTNDSKAFNGTNYPASQRDMRIGVYGVLGLAQGVFVLMANLLSAHGSTHASNILHRQLLNNILQAPMSFFDT
TPTGRIVNRFAGDISTVDDTLPQSLRSWILCFLGIVSTLVMICTATPVFIIVIIPLSIIYVSIQIFYVATSRQLKRLD
SVTRSPIYSHFSETVSGLSVIRAFEHQQRFLKHNEVGIDTNQKCVFSWIVSNRWLAVRLELIGNLIVFFSSLMMVIYK
ATLSGDTVGFVLSNALNITQTLNWLVRMTSEIETNIVAVERINEYIKVENEAPWVTDKRPPPGWPSKGEIRFNNYQVR
YRPELDLVLRGITCDIRSMEKIGVVGRTGAGKSSLTNGLFRILEAAGGQIIIDGVDIASIGLHDLREKLTIIPQDPIL
FSGSLRMNLDPFNHYSDGEIWKALELAHLKTFVAGLQLGLSHEVAEAGDNLSIGQRQLLCLARALLRKSKILIMDEAT
AAVDLETDHLIQMTIQREFSHCTTITIAHRLHTIMDSDKIIVLDNGKIVEYGSPQELLRNSGPFYLMAKEAGIENVNS

```
TSF" } ,
    annot {
      {
        data
          ftable {
            {
              data
                prot {
                  name {
                    "multidrug resistance protein 2" } ,
                  activity {
                    "drug conjugate transporter" } } ,
              location
                whole
                  gi 15130910 } } } } } ,
    annot {
      {
        data
          ftable {
            {
              data
                cdregion {
                  frame one ,
                  code {
                    id 1 } } ,
              comment "alternative splicing" ,
              product
                whole
                  gi 15130910 ,
              location
                int {
                  from 2 ,
                  to 4636 ,
                  id
                    gi 15130909 } ,
              exp-ev experimental } } } } }
```

EMBL

The EMBL format was developed by the EBI, and is used by several major databases including EMBL and SwissProt. Like the GenBank format, this is a human readable informational format and is not geared toward parsing, however, the structure is more regular than that of GenBank, and thus is potentially easier to deal with programmatically.

The EMBL format is line-based and consists of a two-letter code followed by three spaces. The information string begins at character six, and continues up to 80 characters. Each line in the record must have a two-letter identifier, including blank lines, with the exception of the sequence section.

The sequence section begins with a sequence header, denoted by a line containing the two-letter code SQ. The header contains information about the sequence composition. The sequence header is followed by a set of sequence lines. The code for a sequence line is two spaces, so in effect the first letter of each sequence line is at position six. Each sequence line can contain up to 60 sequence characters, grouped into six groups of 10 characters, each group separated by a space. A numeric indication of how many characters of the sequence have been included finishes the line right justified to position 80.

An EMBL record is finished by the two letter code // (similar to the Gen-Bank delimiter).

A complete guide to the EMBL format, including all possible two letter codes, can be found at www.ebi.ac.uk/embl/Documentation/User_manual/format.html

```
ID   TRBG361     standard; RNA; PLN; 1859 BP.
XX
AC   X56734; S46826;
XX
SV   X56734.1
XX
DT   12-SEP-1991 (Rel. 29, Created)
DT   15-MAR-1999 (Rel. 59, Last updated, Version 9)
XX
DE   Trifolium repens mRNA for non-cyanogenic beta-glucosidase
XX
KW   beta-glucosidase.
XX
OS   Trifolium repens (white clover)
OC   Eukaryota; Viridiplantae; Streptophyta; Embryophyta; Tracheophyta;
OC   euphyllophytes; Spermatophyta; Magnoliophyta; eudicotyledons; Rosidae;
OC   Fabales; Fabaceae; Papilionoideae; Trifolium.
XX
RN   [5]
RP   1-1859
RA   Oxtoby E., Dunn M.A., Pancoro A., Hughes M.A.;
RT   "Nucleotide and derived amino acid sequence of the cyanogenic
RT   beta-glucosidase (linamarase) from white clover (Trifolium repens L.).";
RL   Plant Mol. Biol. 17:209-219(1991).
XX
RN   [6]
RP   1-1859
RA   Hughes M.A.;
RT   ;
RL   Submitted (19-NOV-1990) to the EMBL/GenBank/DDBJ databases.
RL   M.A. Hughes, UNIVERSITY OF NEWCASTLE UPON TYNE, MEDICAL SCHOOL, NEW
RL   CASTLE UPON TYNE, NE2  4HH, UK
XX
DR   AGIS; X56734; 17-SEP-1999.
DR   MENDEL; 11000; TRIrp;1162;1.
DR   SWISS-PROT; P26204; BGLS_TRIRP.
XX
FH   Key             Location/Qualifiers
FH
FT   source          1..1859
FT                   /organism="Trifolium repens"
FT                   /db_xref="taxon:3899"
FT                   /tissue_type="leaves"
FT                   /clone_lib="lambda gt10"
FT                   /clone="TRE361"
FT   CDS             14..1495
FT                   /db_xref="MENDEL:11000"
FT                   /db_xref="SWISS-PROT:P26204"
FT                   /note="non-cyanogenic"
FT                   /EC_number="3.2.1.21"
FT                   /product="beta-glucosidase"
FT                   /protein_id="CAA40058.1"
FT                   /translation="MDFIVAIFALFVISSFTITSTNAVEASTLLDIGNLSRSSFPRGFI
FT                   FGAGSSAYQFEGAVNEGGRGPSIWDTFTHKYPEKIRDGSNADITVDQYHRYKEDVGIMK
FT                   DQNMDSYRFSISWPRILPKGKLSGGINHEGIKYYNNLINELLANGIQPFVTLFHWDLPQ
FT                   VLEDEYGGFLNSGVINDFRDYTDLCFKEFGDRVRYWSTLNEPWVFSNSGYALGTNAPGR
FT                   CSASNVAKPGDSGTGPYIVTHNQILAHAEAVHVYKTKYQAYQKGKIGITLVSNWLMPLD
FT                   DNSIPDIKAAERSLDFQFGLFMEQLTTGDYSKSMRRIVKNRLPKFSKFESSLVNGSFDF
```

```
FT                       IGINYYSSSYISNAPSHGNAKPSYSTNPMTNISFEKHGIPLGPRAASIWIYVYPYMFIQ
FT                       EDFEIFCYILKINITILQFSITENGMNEFNDATLPVEEALLNTYRIDYYYRHLYYIRSA
FT                       IRAGSNVKGFYAWSFLDCNEWFAGFTVRFGLNFVD"
FT      mRNA             1..1859
FT                       /evidence=EXPERIMENTAL
XX
SQ      Sequence 1859 BP; 609 A; 314 C; 355 G; 581 T; 0 other;
        aaacaaacca aatatggatt ttattgtagc catatttgct ctgtttgtta ttagctcatt        60
        cacaattact tccacaaatg cagttgaagc ttctactctt cttgacatag gtaacctgag       120
        tcggagcagt tttcctcgtg gcttcatctt tggtgctgga tcttcagcat accaatttga       180
        aggtgcagta aacgaaggcg gtagaggacc aagtatttgg gataccttca cccataaata       240
        tccagaaaaa ataagggatg gaagcaatgc agacatcacg gttgaccaat atcaccgcta       300
        caaggaagat gttgggatta tgaaggatca aaatatggat tcgtatagat tctcaatctc       360
        ttggccaaga atactcccaa agggaaagtt gagcggaggc ataaatcacg aaggaatcaa       420
        atattacaac aaccttatca acgaactatt ggctaacggt atacaaccat ttgtaactct       480
        ttttcattgg gatcttcccc aagtcttaga agatgagtat ggtggtttct taaactccgg       540
        tgtaataaat gattttcgag actatacgga tctttgcttc aaggaatttg gagatagagt       600
        gaggtattgg agtactctaa atgagccatg ggtgtttagc aattctggat atgcactagg       660
        aacaaatgca ccaggtcgat gttcggcctc caacgtggcc aagcctggtg attctggaac       720
        aggaccttat atagttacac acaatcaaat tcttgctcat gcagaagctg tacatgtgta       780
        taagactaaa taccaggcat atcaaaaggg aaagataggc ataacgttgg tatctaactg       840
        gttaatgcca cttgatgata atagcatacc agatataaag gctgccgaga gatcacttga       900
        cttccaattt ggattgttta tggaacaatt aacaacagga gattattcta agagcatgcg       960
        gcgtatagtt aaaaaccgat tacctaagtt ctcaaaattc gaatcaagcc tagtgaatgg      1020
        ttcatttgat tttattggta taaactatta ctcttctagt tatattagca atgcccccttc     1080
        acatggcaat gccaaaccca gttactcaac aaatcctatg accaatattt catttgaaaa      1140
        acatgggata cccttaggtc caagggctgc ttcaatttgg atatatgttt atccatatat      1200
        gtttatccaa gaggacttcg agatcttttg ttacatatta aaaataaata taacaatcct      1260
        gcaattttca atcactgaaa atggtatgaa tgaattcaac gatgcaacac ttccagtaga      1320
        agaagctctt ttgaatactt acagaattga ttactattac cgtcacttat actacattcg      1380
        ttctgcaatc agggctggct caaatgtgaa gggttttttac gcatggtcat ttttggactg     1440
        taatgaatgg tttgcaggct ttactgttcg ttttggatta aactttgtag attagaaaga      1500
        tggattaaaa aggtacccta agctttctgc ccaatggtac aagaactttc tcaaaagaaa      1560
        ctagctagta ttattaaaag aactttgtag tagattacag tacatcgttt gaagttgagt      1620
        tggtgcacct aattaaataa aagaggttac tcttaacata tttttaggcc attcgttgtg      1680
        aagttgttag gctgttattt ctattatact atgttgtagt aataagtgca ttgttgtacc      1740
        agaagctatg atcataacta taggttgatc cttcatgtat cagtttgatg ttgagaatac      1800
        tttgaattaa aagtcttttt ttattttttt aaaaaaaaaa aaaaaaaaaa aaaaaaaa        1859
//
```

PDB

The Protein Data Bank contains information regarding the three-dimensional structure of proteins. A PDB record consists of 12 sections that range from descriptive titles and remarks to structure descriptions, including the atomic coordinates.

Positions 1 through 6 of each line contains a line identifier. Positions 9 and 10 is the continuation marker, and positions 11 through 70 are the actual data, formatted according to the line identifier. Line identifiers must be in a particular order.

Each PDB record ends with a line containing the line identifier END.

A comprehensive guide to the PDB file format is at www.rcsb.org/pdb/docs/format/pdbguide2.2/guide2.2_frame.html

(Note: Several pages of similar lines have been cut out of the REMARK, ATOM, and HETATM sections in the interest of space.)

```
HEADER    OXYGEN STORAGE/TRANSPORT                    13-DEC-99   1DM1
TITLE     2.0 A CRYSTAL STRUCTURE OF THE DOUBLE MUTANT H(E7)V, T(E10)
TITLE     2 R OF MYOGLOBIN FROM APLYSIA LIMACINA
COMPND    MOL_ID: 1;
COMPND    2 MOLECULE: MYOGLOBIN;
COMPND    3 CHAIN: A;
COMPND    4 ENGINEERED: YES;
COMPND    5 MUTATION: YES
SOURCE    MOL_ID: 1;
SOURCE    2 ORGANISM_SCIENTIFIC: APLYSIA LIMACINA;
SOURCE    3 ORGANISM_COMMON: SLUG SEA HARE;
SOURCE    4 EXPRESSION_SYSTEM: ESCHERICHIA COLI;
SOURCE    5 EXPRESSION_SYSTEM_COMMON: BACTERIA
KEYWDS    GLOBIN FOLD
EXPDTA    X-RAY DIFFRACTION
AUTHOR    L.FEDERICI,C.SAVINO,R.MUSTO,C.TRAVAGLINI-ALLOCATELLI,
AUTHOR    2 F.CUTRUZZOLA,M.BRUNORI
REVDAT    1    21-JUN-00 1DM1       0
JRNL          AUTH   L.FEDERICI,C.SAVINO,R.MUSTO,
JRNL          AUTH 2 C.TRAVAGLINI-ALLOCATELLI,F.CUTRUZZOLA,M.BRUNORI
JRNL          TITL   ENGINEERING HIS(E7) AFFECTS THE CONTROL OF HEME
JRNL          TITL 2 REACTIVITY IN APLYSIA LIMACINA MYOGLOBIN
JRNL          REF    BIOCHEM.BIOPHYS.RES.COMM.    V. 269      58 2000
JRNL          REFN   ASTM BBRCA9   US ISSN 0006-291X
REMARK    1
REMARK    2
REMARK    2 RESOLUTION. 1.99 ANGSTROMS.
REMARK    3
REMARK    3 REFINEMENT.
REMARK    3    PROGRAM     : REFMAC
REMARK    3    AUTHORS     : MURSHUDOV,VAGIN,DODSON
REMARK    3
REMARK    3    DATA USED IN REFINEMENT.
REMARK    3    RESOLUTION RANGE HIGH (ANGSTROMS) : 1.99
REMARK    3    RESOLUTION RANGE LOW  (ANGSTROMS) : 59.8
REMARK    3    DATA CUTOFF          (SIGMA(F)) : 2.000
REMARK    3    COMPLETENESS FOR RANGE      (%) : 97.7
REMARK    3    NUMBER OF REFLECTIONS        : 18677
REMARK    3
REMARK    3    FIT TO DATA USED IN REFINEMENT.
REMARK    3    CROSS-VALIDATION METHOD         : NULL
REMARK    3    FREE R VALUE TEST SET SELECTION : RANDOM
REMARK    3    R VALUE     (WORKING + TEST SET) : NULL
REMARK    3    R VALUE         (WORKING SET) : 0.189
REMARK    3    FREE R VALUE                 : 0.216
REMARK    3    FREE R VALUE TEST SET SIZE   (%) : NULL
REMARK    3    FREE R VALUE TEST SET COUNT     : 953
REMARK    3
REMARK    3    NUMBER OF NON-HYDROGEN ATOMS USED IN REFINEMENT.
REMARK    3    PROTEIN ATOMS           : 1079
REMARK    3    NUCLEIC ACID ATOMS      : 0
REMARK    3    HETEROGEN ATOMS         : 43
REMARK    3    SOLVENT ATOMS           : 77
REMARK    3
REMARK    3    B VALUES.
REMARK    3    FROM WILSON PLOT        (A**2) : 29.81
REMARK    3    MEAN B VALUE      (OVERALL, A**2) : NULL
REMARK    3    OVERALL ANISOTROPIC B VALUE.
REMARK    3    B11 (A**2) : NULL
REMARK    3    B22 (A**2) : NULL
REMARK    3    B33 (A**2) : NULL
REMARK    3    B12 (A**2) : NULL
REMARK    3    B13 (A**2) : NULL
REMARK    3    B23 (A**2) : NULL
REMARK    3
REMARK    3    ESTIMATED OVERALL COORDINATE ERROR.
```

```
REMARK   3    ESU BASED ON R VALUE                           (A): NULL
REMARK   3    ESU BASED ON FREE R VALUE                      (A): NULL
REMARK   3    ESU BASED ON MAXIMUM LIKELIHOOD                (A): NULL
REMARK   3    ESU FOR B VALUES BASED ON MAXIMUM LIKELIHOOD (A**2): NULL
REMARK   3
...
DBREF  1DM1 A    1   146  SWS    P02210   GLB_APLLI         1    146
SEQADV 1DM1 ASN A   22  SWS    P02210    ASP    22 CONFLICT
SEQADV 1DM1 HIS A   63  SWS    P02210    VAL    63 ENGINEERED
SEQADV 1DM1 THR A   66  SWS    P02210    ARG    66 ENGINEERED
SEQADV 1DM1 ASN A   80  SWS    P02210    ASP    80 CONFLICT
SEQRES   1 A  146  SER LEU SER ALA ALA GLU ALA ASP LEU ALA GLY LYS SER
SEQRES   2 A  146  TRP ALA PRO VAL PHE ALA ASN LYS ASN ALA ASN GLY ASP
SEQRES   3 A  146  ALA PHE LEU VAL ALA LEU PHE GLU LYS PHE PRO ASP SER
SEQRES   4 A  146  ALA ASN PHE PHE ALA ASP PHE LYS GLY LYS SER VAL ALA
SEQRES   5 A  146  ASP ILE LYS ALA SER PRO LYS LEU ARG ASP HIS SER SER
SEQRES   6 A  146  THR ILE PHE THR ARG LEU ASN GLU PHE VAL ASN ASN ALA
SEQRES   7 A  146  ALA ASN ALA GLY LYS MET SER ALA MET LEU SER GLN PHE
SEQRES   8 A  146  ALA LYS GLU HIS VAL GLY PHE GLY VAL GLY SER ALA GLN
SEQRES   9 A  146  PHE GLU ASN VAL ARG SER MET PHE PRO GLY PHE VAL ALA
SEQRES  10 A  146  SER VAL ALA ALA PRO PRO ALA GLY ALA ASP ALA ALA TRP
SEQRES  11 A  146  THR LYS LEU PHE GLY LEU ILE ILE ASP ALA LEU LYS ALA
SEQRES  12 A  146  ALA GLY LYS
HET    HEM  A 148      43
HETNAM     HEM PROTOPORPHYRIN IX CONTAINING FE
HETSYN     HEM HEME
FORMUL   2  HEM    C34 H32 N4 O4 FE1
FORMUL   3  HOH   *77(H2 O1)
HELIX    1   1 SER A    3  ALA A   15  1                                13
HELIX    2   2 TRP A   14  ASN A   20  1                                 7
HELIX    3   3 ASN A   20  PHE A   36  1                                17
HELIX    4   4 PRO A   37  PHE A   43  5                                 7
HELIX    5   5 SER A   50  SER A   57  1                                 8
HELIX    6   6 PRO A   58  ASN A   77  1                                20
HELIX    7   7 ASN A   80  PHE A   98  1                                19
HELIX    8   8 GLY A  101  ALA A  120  1                                20
HELIX    9   9 GLY A  125  ALA A  144  1                                20
LINK         NE2 HIS A  95                 FE   HEM A 148
CRYST1   89.730   89.730   92.080  90.00  90.00 120.00 H 3         9
ORIGX1      1.000000  0.000000  0.000000        0.00000
ORIGX2      0.000000  1.000000  0.000000        0.00000
ORIGX3      0.000000  0.000000  1.000000        0.00000
SCALE1      0.011140  0.006430  0.000000        0.00000
SCALE2      0.000000  0.012870  0.000000        0.00000
SCALE3      0.000000  0.000000  0.010860        0.00000
ATOM        1  N   SER A   1     -15.388  34.621   9.714  1.00 36.31           N
ATOM        2  CA  SER A   1     -16.267  33.765  10.549  1.00 34.51           C
ATOM        3  C   SER A   1     -17.315  34.569  11.280  1.00 31.49           C
ATOM        4  O   SER A   1     -17.405  35.778  11.189  1.00 31.79           O
ATOM        5  CB  SER A   1     -15.355  33.015  11.504  1.00 38.50           C
ATOM        6  OG  SER A   1     -14.809  34.027  12.355  1.00 41.88           O
...
ATOM     1060  N   ALA A 143     -12.491  36.859  -3.851  1.00 51.73           N
ATOM     1061  CA  ALA A 143     -11.080  36.602  -3.643  1.00 53.40           C
ATOM     1062  C   ALA A 143     -10.604  35.525  -4.583  1.00 54.69           C
ATOM     1063  O   ALA A 143      -9.452  35.598  -4.993  1.00 55.80           O
ATOM     1064  CB  ALA A 143     -10.791  36.265  -2.201  1.00 52.67           C
ATOM     1065  N   ALA A 144     -11.377  34.516  -4.946  1.00 55.40           N
ATOM     1066  CA  ALA A 144     -10.926  33.479  -5.842  1.00 55.53           C
ATOM     1067  C   ALA A 144     -11.133  33.784  -7.312  1.00 56.70           C
ATOM     1068  O   ALA A 144     -10.857  32.896  -8.103  1.00 56.62           O
ATOM     1069  CB  ALA A 144     -11.552  32.143  -5.496  1.00 55.24           C
ATOM     1070  N   GLY A 145     -11.530  34.962  -7.724  1.00 59.00           N
ATOM     1071  CA  GLY A 145     -11.669  35.308  -9.105  1.00 61.97           C
ATOM     1072  C   GLY A 145     -12.911  36.008  -9.579  1.00 63.99           C
ATOM     1073  O   GLY A 145     -12.830  36.905 -10.431  1.00 65.00           O
```

```
ATOM    1074  N    LYS A 146      -14.091  35.629  -9.099  1.00 64.19           N
ATOM    1075  CA   LYS A 146      -15.322  36.222  -9.559  1.00 64.34           C
ATOM    1076  C    LYS A 146      -16.395  36.239  -8.483  1.00 64.47           C
ATOM    1077  O    LYS A 146      -17.330  37.043  -8.641  1.00 62.43           O
ATOM    1078  CB   LYS A 146      -15.891  35.393 -10.706  1.00 65.74           C
ATOM    1079  OXT  LYS A 146      -16.548  35.081  -8.007  1.00 65.43           O
TER     1080       LYS A 146
HETATM  1081  FE   HEM A 148      -22.928  24.481  -5.217  1.00 27.15           FE
HETATM  1082  CHA  HEM A 148      -21.582  21.644  -6.456  1.00 26.05           C
HETATM  1083  CHB  HEM A 148      -22.512  23.374  -2.023  1.00 21.75           C
HETATM  1084  CHC  HEM A 148      -24.868  27.059  -4.010  1.00 24.16           C
HETATM  1085  CHD  HEM A 148      -23.566  25.524  -8.437  1.00 25.14           C
HETATM  1086  N A  HEM A 148      -22.280  22.848  -4.410  1.00 25.05           N
HETATM  1087  C1A  HEM A 148      -21.620  21.819  -5.091  1.00 28.58           C
HETATM  1088  C2A  HEM A 148      -21.006  20.953  -4.149  1.00 28.10           C
HETATM  1089  C3A  HEM A 148      -21.247  21.431  -2.933  1.00 27.03           C
HETATM  1090  C4A  HEM A 148      -22.038  22.606  -3.062  1.00 26.39           C
HETATM  1091  CMA  HEM A 148      -20.780  20.820  -1.594  1.00 25.84           C
HETATM  1092  CAA  HEM A 148      -20.188  19.696  -4.558  1.00 30.74           C
...
HETATM  1189  O    HOH    66      -14.548  22.539  -9.033  1.00 43.11           O
HETATM  1190  O    HOH    67      -42.832  25.949  -6.968  1.00 66.87           O
HETATM  1191  O    HOH    68      -32.642  36.212  19.553  1.00 53.03           O
HETATM  1192  O    HOH    69      -36.051  14.706  11.812  1.00 69.78           O
HETATM  1193  O    HOH    70      -30.164  38.981  18.542  1.00 67.72           O
HETATM  1194  O    HOH    71      -25.116  18.344  12.468  1.00 59.17           O
HETATM  1195  O    HOH    72      -27.237  26.868  17.991  1.00 71.83           O
HETATM  1196  O    HOH    73      -32.897  11.306  -0.328  1.00 63.11           O
HETATM  1197  O    HOH    74      -29.880  13.703   9.080  1.00 30.00           O
HETATM  1198  O    HOH    75      -40.689  29.090   1.181  1.00 30.00           O
HETATM  1199  O    HOH    76      -42.031  31.123  -6.241  1.00 30.00           O
HETATM  1200  O    HOH    77      -33.064  26.126 -17.339  1.00 30.00           O
CONECT   721 1081
CONECT  1081  721 1086 1097 1105
CONECT  1081 1113
CONECT  1082 1087 1117
CONECT  1083 1090 1098
CONECT  1084 1101 1106
CONECT  1085 1109 1114
CONECT  1086 1081 1087 1090
CONECT  1087 1082 1086 1088
CONECT  1088 1087 1089 1092
CONECT  1089 1088 1090 1091
CONECT  1090 1083 1086 1089
CONECT  1091 1089
CONECT  1092 1088 1093
CONECT  1093 1092 1094
CONECT  1094 1093 1095 1096
CONECT  1095 1094
CONECT  1096 1094
CONECT  1097 1081 1098 1101
CONECT  1098 1083 1097 1099
CONECT  1099 1098 1100 1102
CONECT  1100 1099 1101 1103
CONECT  1101 1084 1097 1100
CONECT  1102 1099
CONECT  1103 1100 1104
CONECT  1104 1103
CONECT  1105 1081 1106 1109
CONECT  1106 1084 1105 1107
CONECT  1107 1106 1108 1110
CONECT  1108 1107 1109 1111
CONECT  1109 1085 1105 1108
CONECT  1110 1107
CONECT  1111 1108 1112
CONECT  1112 1111
```

```
CONECT 1113 1081 1114 1117
CONECT 1114 1085 1113 1115
CONECT 1115 1114 1116 1118
CONECT 1116 1115 1117 1119
CONECT 1117 1082 1113 1116
CONECT 1118 1115
CONECT 1119 1116 1120
CONECT 1120 1119 1121
CONECT 1121 1120 1122 1123
CONECT 1122 1121
CONECT 1123 1121
MASTER       267    0    1    9    0    0    0    6 1199    1   45   12
END
```

Fasta

The Fasta file format is the standard format for interchanging simple sequence data. A Fasta record consists of a header line and the sequence. The header, also known as the defline, begins with the > symbol and contains information about the sequence. The sequence is in a multiline format, 70 characters per line.

Any number of Fasta records can be placed in a single file. No special record separator is defined: the > symbol at the beginning of a defline indicates the start of a new record. A file with multiple Fasta records is also referred to as a Fasta library. Sequence types (protein, DNA, or RNA) should not be mixed in Fasta libraries.

Typically, Fasta records have .fa as a file extension. Fasta libraries have .falib as a file extension.

```
>Canis familiaris mRNA for multidrug resistance protein 2 (mrp2 gene)
TCATGCTGGAGAAGTTCTGCAACTCTACGTTTTGGAACTCTTCATTCTTGGATAGCCCAGAAGCGGACCT
GCCACTTTGTTTTGAGCAAACTGTTCTGGTGTGGATTCCCTTGGGTTTCCTTTGGCTCCTGGCCCCTTGG
CAGCTTCTTCATGTGTATAGGACCAAGATCAAGAGATCTTCTATAACCAAACTCTACCTTGCTAAGCAGG
TGCTTGTTGGGTTTCTTCTTATTCTAGCAGCCATAGAGCTGGTCCTTGTACTCACAGAAGACTCTGGAGA
AGCCACAGTCCCCGCCATTAGATACACCAATCCAAGCCTTTACCTGGGCACATGGCTCCTGGTTTTGCTG
ATCCAATACAGCAGGCGATGGTGTGTACAGAAGGATTCTTGGTTCCTGTCTCTATTCTGGATTCTCTCAA
TACTCTGTGGTAGTTTCCAATTTCAGACTCTGATCCGGACACTCTTAAAGGACAGCAATTCTAACTTGGC
TTACTCCTGCCTGTTCTTCATCGGCTATGCACTACAGATCCTGGTCCTGATCCTATCAGCATTTTCAGAA
AAAGATGCCTCCTCAAATAATCCATCATTCACGGCCTCATTTCTGAGTAGCATTACGTTTAGTTGGTATG
ACAGCATTGTTATGAAAGGCTACAAGCAACCTCTGACACTGGAAGATGTGTGGGATGTTGATGAACAGAT
TACAACCAAGGCACTGGTCAGCAAGTTTGAAAAATATATGGTAGAAGAGCTGCAGAAGGCCAGAAAGACC
CTCCAGAAACAGCAACAGAGGAACACCCAGGGGAAGTCTGGAGAAAGGCTGCATGACTTGAACAAGAATC
AGAGTCAAAGCCAAGATATCCTTGTTCTGGAAGAAGTTAAAAAGAAAAAAAAGAAGTCTGGGACCACAGA
AAAGTTTCCCAAGTCCTGGTTGGTCAAGAGTCTCTTCAAAACTTTCTATGTCATACTCTTGAAATCATTC
CTACTGAAGCTGGTGTTTGACCTTCTCACGTTCCTGAATCCTCAGCTGCTGAAGTTGCTGATCTCCTTTG
CAAATGACCCAGACATGTATGTGTGGACTGGGTATTTCTATTCGGTCCTCTTCTTTGTTGGTGGCTCTCAT
CCAGTCTCTCTGCCTTCAGAGCTACTTTCAAATGTGCTTCATGTTGGGTGTAAACGTACGGACAACCATC
ATGGCTTCCATATACAAGAAGGCGCTGACCCTTTCCAACCAGGCCAGGAAGCAGTACACCATTGGAGAAA
CAGTGAACCTGATGTCTGTGGATGCTCAGAAGCTCATGGATGTGACCAACTTCATTCATCTGCTGTGGTC
AAATGTTCTCCAGATTGCTTTATCTATCTACTTCCTGTGGGCAGAGCTGGGACCCTCCATCTTAGCAGGT
GTTGGGGTGATGATACTCCTAATTCCAGTTAATGGGCTACTTGCCTCTAAGAGTAGAGCTATTCAGGTAA
AAAATATGAAGAATAAAGACAAACGTTTAAAGATCATGAATGAAATTCTCAGTGGGATCAAGATCCTGAA
ATATTTTGCCTGGGAACCTTCATTCAAAAACCAAGTCCACGAACTTCGGAAGAAAGAGCTCAAGAACCTG
CTGACCTTCGGGCAGATGCAGTCTGTAATGGTGTTTCTCTTATACTTAACTCCGGTCTTGGTGTCTGTGA
TCACGTTTTCAGTTTACACTCTGGTGGACAGCAATAATGTTTTGGATGCAGAGAAGGCATTCACCTCCAT
```

```
CACCCTCTTCAATATCCTGCGCTTTCCCCTAAGCATGCTCCCCATGGTAATCTCCTCACTGCTCCAGGCC
AGCGTTTCCAGAGAACGCCTGGAAAAGTACTTGGGAGGGGATGACTTAGACACATCCGCCATTCGACGTG
ACAGCAGTTCTGACAAAGCTGTGCAGTTCTCAGAGGCCTCCTTCACCTGGGACCGGGACTCGGAAGCCAC
AATCCGAGATGTGAACCTGGAGATTATGCCAGGCCTTATGGTGGCTGTGGTGGGCACTGTAGGCTCTGGG
AAGTCTTCCTTGATGTCAGCCATGCTGGGAGAAATGGAAGATGTCCATGGGCACATCACCATCAAGGGCA
CCATAGCCTACGTCCCACAGCAATCCTGGATTCAGAATGGCACCATAAAGGACAACATCCTTTTTGGATC
CGAGTTGGATGAAAAGAGATACCAGCAGGTGCTAGAAGCCTGTGCCCTCCTACCAGACTTGGAAGTGCTG
CCGGGAGGAGACCTGGCTGAGATTGGAGAGAAGGGTATAAATCTTAGTGGGGGTCAGAAGCAGCGGATTA
GCCTGGCCAGAGCTACCTATCAGAATTCAGACATCTATGTTCTGGATGACCCCCTGTCAGCTGTGGATGC
TCATGTGGGAAGACATATTTTCAATAAGGTCTTGGGTCCCAATGGCCTATTGAAAGGCAAGACTCGTCTC
TTGGTTACACATAGCATTCACTTTCTTCCCCAAGTGGATGAGATTGTGGTTCTGGGGAATGGCACCATCT
TGGAGAAGGGATCCTACAACACTCTGCTGGCCAAGAAAGGATTGTTTGCTAAGATTCTGAAGGCATTCAC
AAAACAGACGGGTCCTGAAGGAGAGGCCACAGTCAATGAGGACAGTGAAGAAGATGATGACTGTGGGCTG
ATGCCCAGTGTGGAGGAAATCCCTGAGGAAGTGGCCTCCTTGACCATGAAAAGAGAGAACAGCCTTCATC
GAACACTTAGTCGCAGTTCCAGGTCCAGGAGCAGACATCAGAAATCCCTAAGAAACTCTTTGAAAACCCG
GAATGTGAACACTCTGAAGGAGGAGGAGGAACCAGTGAAAGGACAAAAACTAATTAAGAAGGAATTCATA
CAAACTGGAAAGGTGAAGTTCTCCATCTACCTGAAGTACCTACGAGCAATAGGATGGTATTTGATATTCC
TCATCATTTTTGCCTATGTGATCAATTCTGTGGCTTATATTGGATCCAACCTCTGGCTCAGTGCTTGGAC
CAATGACTCTAAAGCCTTTAATGGCACTAACTATCCAGCCTCTCAGAGGGACATGAGAATTGGCGTCTAT
GGAGTTCTGGGATTAGCTCAAGGTGTGTTTGTGCTCATGGCAAATCTCTTGAGTGCCCATGGTTCCACCC
ATGCATCAAACATCCTTCACAGGCAACTGCTAAACAACATCCTTCAAGCACCCATGAGTTTTTTTGACAC
AACACCCACAGGTCGGATTGTGAACAGGTTTGCTGGTGATATTTCCACAGTGGATGACACCCTCCCCCAA
TCCTTGCGCAGCTGGATATTGTGTTTCCTGGGAATAGTCAGCACTCTTGTCATGATCTGCACGGCCACTC
CAGTGTTCATCATCGTCATCATTCCTCTTAGCATTATTTATGTGTCTATTCAGATATTTTATGTGGCTAC
TTCCCGCCAGCTGAAACGTCTAGACTCTGTCACCAGATCCCCAATTTACTCTCACTTCAGTGAGACAGTG
TCAGGTTTGTCCGTCATCCGTGCCTTTGAGCATCAGCAGAGATTTCTGAAACACAATGAAGTGGGGATTG
ACACCAACCAGAAATGTGTCTTTTCCTGGATTGTCTCCAACAGATGGCTTGCAGTTCGTCTGGAGCTGAT
TGGGAACTTGATTGTCTTCTTTTCATCCCTGATGATGGTTATTTATAAAGCTACCCTAAGTGGAGACACT
GTGGGCTTTGTTCTGTCCAATGCACTTAATATCACACAGACCCTGAACTGGCTAGTGAGGATGACGTCAG
AAATAGAGACCAACATTGTGGCTGTTGAAAGAATAAATGAATACATAAAAGTGGAAAATGAGGCACCCTG
GGTGACTGATAAGAGACCTCCCCCAGGTTGGCCCAGCAAAGGGGAGATTCGGTTTAACAACTACCAAGTG
CGGTACCGGCCTGAACTGGATCTTGTACTGAGAGGGATCACTTGTGATATTAGGAGCATGGAGAAGATTG
GTGTGGTGGGCAGAACAGGAGCTGGGAAGTCATCCTTGACAAATGGCCTCTTCAGAATCCTAGAGGCTGC
AGGTGGTCAGATCATCATTGATGGGGTAGATATTGCTTCCATTGGGCTCCATGACCTCCGAGAAAAATTG
ACCATCATCCCCCAGGATCCCATCCTGTTCTCTGGAAGCCTGAGGATGAATCTAGACCCTTTTAACCACT
ACTCAGATGGGGAGATTTGGAAGGCCTTGGAGCTGGCTCACCTCAAAACATTTGTGGCTGGCCTGCAACT
GGGGTTGTCCCACGAAGTGGCAGAGGCTGGTGACAACCTTAGCATAGGGCAGAGGCAGCTACTGTGCCTG
GCCAGGGCTCTGCTTCGGAAATCCAAGATTCTGATCATGGATGAGGCCACTGCTGCGGTGGACCTAGAGA
CCGATCACCTCATCCAGATGACCATCCAAAGGGAGTTCTCCCACTGCACGACTATCACCATTGCTCACAG
GCTACACACCATCATGGACAGTGACAAGATAATAGTCCTAGACAATGGGAAGATTGTAGAGTATGGCAGC
CCTCAAGAACTGCTGAGAAATTCGGGCCCCTTTTATTTGATGGCCAAAGAAGCTGGCATTGAAAATGTGA
ACAGCACATCGTTCTGACAGTAGGTCCCATGGGCTGAAAAAAGGACTATAAGATCATTCCTTATTTTTTG
TGAGAGATACTACACAGAAGTTTGTAAAATATACATTTTTGAAGAAGGATTGTTATATCCAGCTACAGCG
GACCACCCCCAATCTTGCTTTGATGATCCCACTTCAATTTTATCTCCTTCATACTTACCTTCCCAGAGAT
AACTAACCTGAATTTTGTGATAATGATATCCTCCTGCTTTTCATTTTAGTTTTACTACTTGGTATGTACC
CTTAAACAAGATATACCTTTTTTAATTTATGTGA
```

BLAST

The BLAST sequence alignment programs were developed to quickly search sequence databases. These programs use several specially formatted files as a search library. A nucleotide search library consists of an index file with the extension. nhr, and two binary files with the extension .nin and .nsq. A protein library consists of the analogous files with extensions .phr, .pin, and .psq.

BLAST libraries are typically produced from Fasta libraries using the formatdb program, available from NCBI. The index file contains the deflines and pointers to the compressed sequences in the binary files.

It is probably worth emphasizing again (from the NCBI formatdb documentation) the following:

DISCLAIMER: The internal structure of the BLAST databases is subject to change with little or no notice. The readdb API should be used to extract data from the BLAST databases. Readdb is part of the NCBI toolkit (ftp://ftp.ncbi.nih.gov/toolbox/ncbi_tools/), readdb.h contains a list of supported function calls.

ACEDB

The ACEBD genome informatics system stores and displays multiple types of genomic data. The data schema is customizable, and the data model is closely integrated into the operation of the system. Data is stored in a set of structured binary files, and the data model specifies a tree for each object class based upon tag-value pairs. The value may either be a specified data type, a sub-tag, or a pointer to another object class.

Data is imported and exported through text files called ace files (from the file extension.ace). The data model is responsible for parsing the text in an ace file to and from the binary file. This renders any ace file parser to be fully dependent upon the model file. Several parsers exist to translate ace files to and from other formats.

Data can also be extracted from ACEDB programmatically using programs like tace and perlace. These programs create a functional interface that respond to ace queries without the overhead of using the X-Windows GUI. More detailed information can be found in the ACEDB documentation library at www.acedb.org.

```
<ace file> ::= <object update>                                          |

<object update> NL NL <ace file>                                        ;

<object update> ::= <class name> <name>
                | <class name> <name> NL <data lines>
                | -D <class name> <name>         /* Delete */
                | -R <class name> <name> <name>  /* Remame */
                | -A <class name> <name> <name>  /* Alias */
                ;

<data lines> ::= <data line>
                | <data line> NL <data lines>
                ;
<data line> ::= <path>
                | -D <path>          /* Deletion */
                | -T <path>          /* Tops within column, not in 1.8 */
                | -R <datum> <path>  /* Substitution, not in 1.8 */
                ;
```

```
<path> ::= <simple path>
         | <simple path> # <path>
           ;
<simple path> ::= <tag>
                | <tag> <data list>
                  ;
<data list> ::= <datum>
              | <datum> <data list>
                ;

<tag> ::= /* string starting with a letter or a digit
                          and containing letters, digits or_' */
          ;
<class name> ::= /* string starting with a letter or a digit
                          and containing letters, digits or_' */
             ;
<datum> ::= /* string  containing letters, digits or_' */
          | " /* arbitrary printable string protected by double quotes */ "
            ;
```

Index

Perl Programming for Biologists,   D. Curtis Jamison
ISBN 0-471-43059-5   Copyright © 2003 Wiley-Liss, Inc.